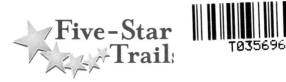

T0356960

West Virginia's
Monongahela
National Forest

Five-Star Trails: West Virginia's Monongahela National Forest
40 Spectacular Hikes in the Allegheny Mountains
1st edition 2000
2nd edition 2006
3rd edition 2017
4th edition 2022
Copyright © 2000, 2006, 2017, and 2022 by Johnny Molloy

Cover design: Scott McGrew
Text design: Annie Long
Front cover photo: Bear Rocks *(See Hike 1, page 20.)* © anthony heflin / Shutterstock
Back cover photo: Spruce Knob and Huckleberry Trail *(See Hike 19, page 101.)* © Johnny Molloy
Interior photos: Johnny Molloy, except where noted
Cartography and elevation profiles: Johnny Molloy and Steve Jones
Project editor: Holly Cross
Proofreader: Vanessa Rusch
Indexer: Rich Carlson

Cataloging-in-Publication Data is available from the Library of Congress.
Names: Molloy, Johnny, 1961– author.
Title: Five-star trails West Virginia's Monongahela National Forest :
    40 spectacular hikes in the Allegheny Mountains / Johnny Molloy.
Other titles: Forty spectacular hikes in the Allegheny Mountains
Description: Fourth Edition. | Birmingham, AL : Menasha Ridge Press, [2022] |
    Series: Five-star trails | Includes index.
Identifiers: LCCN 2021057538 (print) | LCCN 2021057539 (ebook) |
    ISBN 9781634043441 (Paperback) | ISBN 9781634043458 (eBook)
Subjects: LCSH: Hiking--West Virginia--Monongahela National Forest—Guidebooks. |
    Trails—West Virginia—Monongahela National Forest—Guidebooks. |
    Monongahela National Forest (W. Va.)—Guidebooks.
Classification: LCC GV199.42.W42 M6655 2022 (print) | LCC GV199.42.W42 (ebook) |
    DDC 796.5109754/5—dc23/eng/20220224
LC record available at https://lccn.loc.gov/2021057538
LC ebook record available at https://lccn.loc.gov/2021057539

 MENASHA RIDGE PRESS
An imprint of AdventureKEEN
2204 First Ave. S., Ste. 102
Birmingham, AL 35233
menasharidgepress.com
800-678-7006; fax 877-374-9016

Visit menasharidge.com for a complete listing of our books and for ordering information. Contact us at our website, at facebook.com/menasharidge, or at twitter.com/menasharidge with questions or comments. To find out more about who we are and what we're doing, visit blog.menasharidge.com.

SAFETY NOTICE Though the author and publisher have made every effort to ensure that the information in this book is accurate at press time, they are not responsible for any loss, damage, injury, or inconvenience that may occur while using this book—you are responsible for your own safety and health on the trail. The fact that a hike is described in this book does not mean that it will be safe for you. Always check local conditions (which can change from day to day), know your own limitations, and consult a map. For information about trail and other closures, check the "Contacts" listings in the hike profiles.

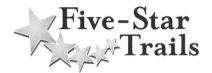

Five-Star Trails

West Virginia's
Monongahela
National Forest

40 Spectacular Hikes in the Allegheny Mountains

4TH EDITION

JOHNNY MOLLOY

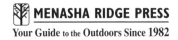

MENASHA RIDGE PRESS
Your Guide to the Outdoors Since 1982

Five-Star Trails: Monongahela National Forest

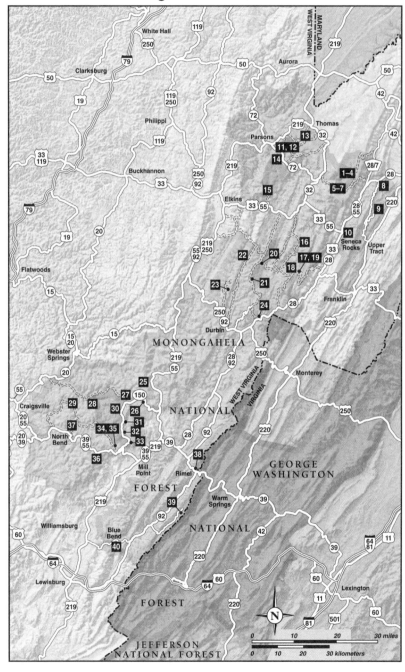

Contents

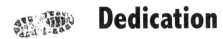

Dedication

This book is for Keri Anne Molloy.

Acknowledgments

Thanks to Oboz for the great hiking shoes and to Kelty and Sierra Designs for the fine sleeping bags, tents, and camping equipment I used all over the frontcountry and backcountry of the Monongahela National Forest. Thanks to my wife, Keri Anne, most of all for hiking and camping with me in this West Virginia paradise.

—*Johnny Molloy*

Preface

The Monongahela National Forest, located entirely within the Mountain State, is the heart and soul of wild, wonderful West Virginia. The numbers are as follows: more than 900,000 acres of land with elevations ranging from 900 to 4,862 feet, including Spruce Knob—the highest point in the state; 600 miles of cold-water fisheries, including 90% of the native brook-trout waters in the state; 130 miles of warm-water fisheries; more than 115,000 acres of designated wilderness; over 75 tree species; and more than 700 miles of marked and maintained hiking trails.

Formed in 1920, the "Mon" is about more than numbers. It is a natural getaway for native mountaineers and outdoors enthusiasts from the Mid-Atlantic metropolises as well as visitors nationwide. And well it should be. Climbers can scale Seneca Rocks. Auto tourists can enjoy the vistas of the Highland Scenic Highway. Mountain bikers can pedal Canaan Mountain. Campers can spend the night at any of the fine campgrounds scattered throughout the national forest. Hikers can enjoy the Mon from the Dolly Sods up north to way down south near Blue Bend.

The first trails were made by American Indians who lived in the valleys of the major rivers here—the Cheat, the Tygart, the Greenbrier, and the Potomac. Pioneers used the same trails, spreading west over the Alleghenies and settling in the fertile valleys.

The high forests remained mostly untouched until after West Virginia became a state during the Civil War. Battles were fought to control passes through the rugged mountains on what later became national forest land. A notable clash was over Cheat Summit Fort, where Robert E. Lee himself failed to wrestle the stronghold from Union hands. On June 20, 1863, the western part of the Old Dominion became the state of West Virginia.

America expanded, and the need for wood grew. The spread of the railroad and use of high-speed band saws opened the mountains of West Virginia to removal of vast stands of virgin woodland. Within 30 years, much of the state was cut over. Then, because there was no vegetation to absorb the slow waters flowing from the mountains, floods submerged the landscape. This watery devastation of the lowlands, particularly the flood of 1907, led to the creation of the Monongahela National Forest. Federal management of these lands resulted in watershed protection among other things.

There was much work to do: replanting trees, cutting roads, and building fire towers and hiking trails. At first, the work was slow. Many mountaineers resented the presence of the feds in their backyard. Ironically, it was the Great Depression that sped the evolution of the national forest. Many young men, unable to find a job, joined the Civilian Conservation Corps, which established work camps throughout the Monongahela. For nearly 10 years they made a mark on the forest. To this day, you can see their handiwork at campgrounds like Blue Bend.

The highlands began to recover. Through wildlife management programs, native species of the Alleghenies began to thrive. White-tailed deer lingered on the edge of clearings; black bears furtively fed on fall's acorns and other natural fare. Other smaller critters, from salamanders to falcons, called the wooded ridges and valleys home. Later, several wildernesses were established to protect unique large swaths of the national forest.

Today, visitors can return to a grand wild land once again to fish for secretive brook trout, to listen to the wind whistle through highland spruce woods, to identify colorful wildflowers, or to see the changing seasons from a magnificent rock vista.

SOUTH FORK FALLS ON SOUTH FORK RED RUN *(See Hike 11, page 64.)*

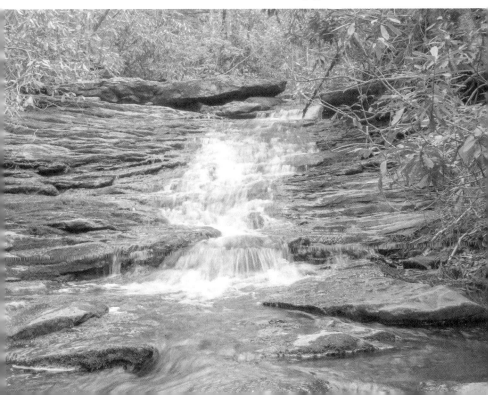

To best enjoy the Mon you must take to your feet. This book details 40 of the Monongahela's best hikes. These hikes head to overlooks, waterfalls, and wildernesses, as well as scenic cultural and historical sites, lakes, and rivers. There are ample rewarding treks, for the Monongahela National Forest is an incredibly attractive land, a place where mountains tower thousands of feet above fertile valleys, where crashing cataracts plunge into deep forests, where rock overlooks and wide meadows deliver resplendent vistas, and where brawling rivers cut deep gorges through majestic highlands.

It is where the Falls of Hills Creek makes its exceptional plunge into a rock cathedral. Along the way to the falls you traverse a rugged gorge. It is where hikers walk regal ridges to expansive vistas. Other trails take you through biological wonderlands such as Cranberry Glades Botanical Area. There, West Virginia's largest tundra wetland harbors rare plants while availing vistas of surrounding mountains.

Speaking of waterfalls, vertical variation and ample rain create an abundance of waterfalls in these parts. In addition to the cataracts already mentioned, there are a host of falls in the Seneca Creek Backcountry, along Red Creek and its tributaries in the Dolly Sods Wilderness, and on lower Otter Creek, deep in the Otter Creek Wilderness. Then add the waterfalls of the Cranberry Wilderness. Big Beechy Run Falls makes its wide drop, the Falls of Middle Fork form a big slide, and interestingly named Hell For Certain Falls dives off a ledge. It is an easy family hike to picturesque Lick Branch Falls. And there are still other, more modest falls. The cascades at the forks of Tea Creek enhance the excellent hiking destination that is the Tea Creek Backcountry. The spillers along the East Fork of the Greenbrier are a less-visited aquatic feature.

Other hikes take you to—and through—historic destinations. The Cowpasture Loop leads to a former federal prison camp without walls, where the isolation and harsh climate discouraged escape. The Camp Five Run Loop takes you by cabins built for early Monongahela National Forest rangers. Those structures are now listed on the National Register of Historic Places. Other trails travel along logging grades from the 1800s and past former logger camps.

And what about hikes for solitude? Take the Laurel Creek Circuit along a mountain stream that ascends to a mountaintop before dropping to the lowlands to complete a loop. The hike up Johns Camp Run and onto Shavers Mountain presents hiking where you can commune with nature one on one. The Gauley Mountain Loop rambles remote reaches of the Monongahela National

Forest, crossing over streams and mountain passes and through bottomland meadows where wildlife may be seen.

And there are still more possibilities included in this guide, places where you can not only hike but also combine trail trekking with other activities in the Monongahela National Forest. The trails of Lake Sherwood Recreation Area take you along a scenic impoundment and to the ridge dividing West Virginia and Virginia, where overlooks extend into both states. Upon returning to Lake Sherwood, you can camp, swim, fish, or picnic. Or walk the loop around Big Bend in Smoke Hole Canyon, then overnight in their campground and paddle the South Branch Potomac River the next morning. Or hike up to Seneca Rocks, take in the wonderful views there, then rock climb or go bouldering in addition to camping at nearby Seneca Shadows Campground. Take the loop around Summit Lake, then camp, fish, or paddle its mountain-rimmed shores.

Who can forget the views to be had on Monongahela hikes? Rohrbaugh Overlook and Blackbird Knob in the incomparable Dolly Sods Wilderness deliver a visual feast, as do panoramas from Chimney Top along North Fork Mountain near Petersburg, from atop Black Mountain, and in multiples from Spruce Knob and the Huckleberry Trail. And how can we leave out the vista from aptly named Table Rock?

Hikes in this book range from under 1 mile to more than 17 miles, creating opportunities for hikers of all ages and abilities. Therefore, the best hikes in the Monongahela National Forest can mean a ramble through the remote highland backcountry, a trek to a crashing cascade, or a quick escape to an eye-popping vista. It all depends on your disposition, company, and desires. So not only is the where to hike component covered, but so is what type of hike. As far as when to go: You can hike year-round in West Virginia (though snow may close access roads to higher destinations), but most people hike from early spring through late fall. However, the varied elevations within the Monongahela National Forest make winter hiking a viable and desirable option. The important thing is getting out there and enjoying the wonderful wild trails and terrain of this scenic slice of the Mountain State.

This variety of hikes reflects the variety of opportunities in the Monongahela National Forest. I sought to include hikes covering routes of multiple lengths, ranging from easy to difficult. Trail configurations are diverse as well—including out-and-back hikes, loops, and balloon loops. Hike settings vary from developed recreation areas to the wildernesses in the back of beyond.

The routes befit a range of abilities and hiking experience. Simply scan the Table of Contents, randomly flip through the book, or utilize the hiking recommendations list on pages xiii–xiv. Find your hike, get out there, and enjoy it. And bring a friend too. Enjoying nature in the company of another is a great way to enhance your relationship as well as escape from the smartphone, television, Internet, and other electronic chains that bind us to the daily grind.

One last thing—there is a reason I live in the shadow of the Appalachians. Having written outdoor guidebooks covering 27 states, I truly believe that these West Virginia highlands comprise one of the best parts of the best country on God's green earth. May this book help you enjoy the wonderful, rewarding trails of the Monongahela National Forest. The Mon is one of West Virginia's special natural resources—it's waiting for you.

—Johnny Molloy

Recommended Hikes

Best for Accessibility

10   Seneca Rocks (p. 59; partial access)
19   Spruce Knob and Huckleberry Trail (p. 101; partial access)
29   Lick Branch Falls (p. 148)
35   Cranberry Glades Interpretive Boardwalk (p. 174)
36   Falls of Hills Creek (p. 178; partial access)
37   Summit Lake Loop (p. 182; partial access)

Best for Dogs

6   Boars Nest Loop (p. 42)
17   North Prong Loop (p. 92)
20   Laurel Fork North Wilderness (p. 105)
23   Shavers Mountain via Johns Camp Run (p. 118)
25   Bear Pen Ridge Loop (p. 130)

Best for History

9   Big Bend Loop (p. 54)
10   Seneca Rocks (p. 59)
21   Camp Five Run Loop (p. 109)
27   Tea Creek Loop (p. 138)
34   Cowpasture Loop (p. 169)

Best for Kids

13   Blackwater Canyon Trail (p. 72)
19   Spruce Knob and Huckleberry Trail (p. 101)
32   Black Mountain Circuit (p. 161)
33   High Rock (p. 165)
35   Cranberry Glades Interpretive Boardwalk (p. 174)
36   Falls of Hills Creek (p. 178)

Best for Nature Lovers

7   Red Creek Plains (p. 46)
11   Canaan Mountain Backcountry Circuit (p. 64)
24   East Fork Greenbrier Hike (p. 123)
31   Tumbling Rock Loop (p. 157)
39   Lake Sherwood Loop (p. 191)

Best for Scenery

2   Blackbird Knob Vista (p. 25)
5   Dunkenbarger Loop (p. 37)
10   Seneca Rocks (p. 59)
34   Cowpasture Loop (p. 169)
39   Lake Sherwood Loop (p. 191)

Best for Seclusion

15   Otter Creek Wilderness Loop (p. 81)
16   Horton–Spring Ridge Loop (p. 88)
23   Shavers Mountain via Johns Camp Run (p. 118)
25   Bear Pen Ridge Loop (p. 130)
38   Laurel Creek Circuit (p. 187)

Best for Views

1   Raven Ridge Loop (p. 20)
4   Rohrbaugh Overlook (p. 33)
8   Chimney Top (p. 50)
12   Table Rock Overlook (p. 68)
19   Spruce Knob and Huckleberry Trail (p. 101)
33   High Rock (p. 165)

Best for Waterfalls

3   Red Creek Falls via Fisher Spring Run (p. 29)
18   Upper Falls of Seneca Creek (p. 96)
22   High Falls (p. 114)

Best for Waterfalls *(continued)*

Best for Water Lovers

Best for Wildflowers

Best for Wildlife

SOAK IN VIEWS LIKE THIS ONE ON THE CHIMNEY TOP HIKE. *(See Hike 8, page 50.)*

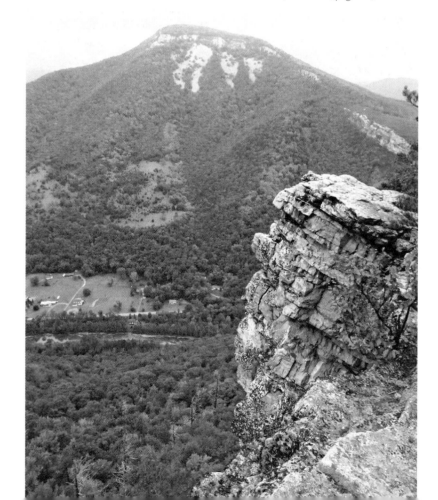

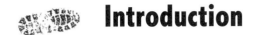 # Introduction

About This Book

Welcome to this new edition of *Five-Star Trails: West Virginia's Monongahela National Forest.* This guide details 40 fantastic hikes in the only national forest entirely in West Virginia, presenting the reader with an array of treks that reflect the magnificence of the area, ranging from the ridges and valleys of the Greenbrier River to the large Cranberry Wilderness, from the lesser-visited Laurel Fork North Wilderness and varied Seneca Creek Backcountry to the Otter Creek Wilderness and splendid Dolly Sods/Roaring Plains area, and the lands between. The vast lands of the Monongahela National Forest are a hiker's nirvana, where trails course throughout the superlative beauty of the Allegheny Highlands. These destinations include developed recreation areas and out-of-the-way, stand-alone trails as well as federally designated wildernesses with elaborate pathway networks.

I assert the Monongahela is one of the best outdoor destinations in the United States. Proximity to seemingly endless outdoor opportunities—hiking, paddling, bicycling, camping, hunting, fishing, nature study, and more—vastly enhance the quality of life here. Hundreds of miles of trails lace these West Virginia mountain lands. The geologically fascinating highlands of the Mountain State lead into deep canyons, wild waterfalls, and unique rock features. Hikes in this book cover destinations throughout the Monongahela National Forest, from the untamed grandeur of the Falls of Hills Creek in the southwest near Richwood to view-laden Blue Bend in the southeast near White Sulphur Springs, to the lofty plateau of Dolly Sods in the northeast near Petersburg, to one of the state's best hiking destinations—Otter Creek Wilderness—to the northwest above Elkins.

Moreover, the West Virginia Appalachians are ideal for hiking because we have four distinct and beautiful seasons. If you like winter, the mountains, regularly rising to more than 4,000 feet, deliver all the snow your average hiker wants. Yet many mild days occur that are perfect for trail trekkers, especially in the lower areas on the eastern side of the national forest, near Virginia. The elevation and terrain variations make spring exciting, too, as the season of rebirth grows its way from the river valleys to the spruce-clad high country. Wildflowers follow. Summer finds many escaping to cool waters and to refreshing mountaintops where heat-relieving breezes blow. During autumn the Monongahela's incredible variety of trees explode in their annual color display brought on by warm, dry days and cool nights.

How do you get started? Peruse this book, pick out a hike, and strike out on the trail. The wide assortment of paths, distances, difficulties, and destinations will suit any hiker's mood and company. Try them all—the varied hikes will leave you appreciating the nature of this region more than you ever imagined.

Monongahela National Forest's Geographic Divisions

The hikes in this book have been divided into three geographic divisions. **Dolly Sods Wilderness–Otter Creek Wilderness Area** covers hikes in the national forest's north region, separated from points south by US 33 that cuts east–west across the forest. The hikes here not only include the inspiring Dolly Sods Wilderness and rugged Otter Creek Wilderness, but also Canaan Mountain Backcountry and along the geologically fascinating North Fork Mountain and crystalline South Branch Potomac River. Hike to elevated open lands, stony ridges, or remote wildernesses.

The **Seneca Creek Backcountry–Laurel Fork Wilderness Area** section includes the section south of US 33 down to where US 250 and WV 28 cross the forest east to west, near Bartow. This swath of land atop Spruce Knob includes the loftiest terrain in the Monongahela and the trail-heavy Seneca Creek Backcountry, where waterfalls, overlooks, and excellent loop hikes await. It is where the Laurel Fork Valley forms the heart of two wildernesses, where scenic rivers and wide-open meadows make for visually stimulating and wildlife-rich terrain.

The **Greater Cranberry Wilderness Area** extends south of the US 250 and WV 28 east–west crossing on the Monongahela down to the east–west I-64 crossing of the Mountain State. This long segment encompasses not only the vast area and trail network that is the Cranberry Wilderness and adjacent Cranberry Backcountry, but also paths of the bordering Highland Scenic Highway and Tea Creek Backcountry, as well as outlier destinations. It is a land rich with waterfalls and places where you can get deep in the wilds, far from civilization. Yet, developed recreation areas such as Summit Lake, Lake Sherwood, and Blue Bend allow fun and rewarding hikes at destinations with facilities ranging from hot showers to campsites to additional recreation pastimes like boating, swimming, and fishing.

Altogether, the trail-laced geographic regions of the Monongahela National Forest create a mosaic of natural splendidness that will please the most discriminating hiker.

How to Use This Guidebook

Overview Map, Regional Maps, and Map Legend

The overview map on page iv depicts the location of the primary trailhead for all 40 of the hikes described in this book. The numbers shown on the overview map pair with the table of contents on the facing page. Each hike's number remains with that hike throughout the book. Thus, if you spot an appealing hiking area on the overview map, you can flip through the book and find those hikes easily by their numbers at the top of the first page for each profile. This book is divided into regions, and prefacing each regional chapter is a regional map. The regional maps provide more detail than the overview map, bringing you closer to the hikes. A legend explaining the map symbols used throughout the book appears below.

Trail Maps

In addition to the overview and regional maps, a detailed map of each hike's route appears with its profile. On this map, symbols indicate the trailhead, the complete route, significant features, facilities, and topographic landmarks such as creeks, overlooks, and peaks.

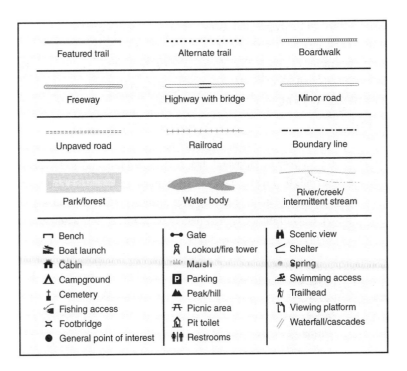

Featured trail	Alternate trail	Boardwalk
Freeway	Highway with bridge	Minor road
Unpaved road	Railroad	Boundary line
Park/forest	Water body	River/creek/ intermittent stream

⌐ Bench	•—• Gate	⋔ Scenic view
⛴ Boat launch	🜊 Lookout/fire tower	⌐ Shelter
♠ Cabin	〰 Marsh	⦿ Spring
▲ Campground	P Parking	⚓ Swimming access
⚑ Cemetery	▲ Peak/hill	⚡ Trailhead
⟜ Fishing access	🕱 Picnic area	⎵ Viewing platform
⋈ Footbridge	🏠 Pit toilet	// Waterfall/cascades
● General point of interest	♦♦ Restrooms	

To produce the highly accurate maps in this book, I used a handheld GPS unit to gather data while hiking each route, and then sent that data to the publisher's expert cartographers. Be aware, though, that your GPS device is no substitute for sound, sensible navigation that takes into account the conditions that you observe while hiking. Further, despite the high quality of the maps in this book, the publisher and I think it wise to carry an additional map, such as the ones noted in each hike profile's introductory listing for "Maps," either on paper or on your smartphone.

Elevation Profile

This diagram represents the rises and falls of the trail as viewed from the side, over the complete distance (in miles) of that trail. On the diagram's vertical axis, or height scale, the number of feet indicated between each tick mark lets you visualize the climb. To avoid making flat hikes look steep and steep hikes appear flat, varying height scales provide an accurate image of each hike's climbing difficulty.

The Hike Profile

This book contains a concise and informative narrative of each hike from beginning to end. The text will get you from a well-known road or highway to the trailhead, through the twists and turns of the hike route, back to the trailhead, and to notable nearby attractions, if there are any. Each profile opens with the route's star ratings, GPS trailhead coordinates, and other key information. Below is an explanation of the introductory elements that give you a snapshot of each of this book's 40 routes.

STAR RATINGS

The hikes in *Five-Star Trails: West Virginia's Monongahela National Forest* were carefully chosen to provide an overall five-star experience, and they represent the diversity of trails found in the region. Each hike was assigned a one- to five-star rating in each of the following categories: scenery, trail condition, suitability for children, level of difficulty, and degree of solitude. Here's how the star ratings for each of the five categories break down:

FOR SCENERY:

★ ★ ★ ★ ★   Unique, picturesque panoramas

★ ★ ★ ★   Diverse vistas

★ ★ ★   Pleasant views

★ ★   Unchanging landscape

★   Not selected for scenery

FOR TRAIL CONDITION:

★ ★ ★ ★ ★   Consistently well maintained

★ ★ ★ ★   Stable, with no surprises

★ ★ ★   Average terrain to negotiate

★ ★   Inconsistent, with good and poor areas

★   Rocky, overgrown, or often muddy

FOR CHILDREN:

★ ★ ★ ★ ★   Babes in strollers are welcome

★ ★ ★ ★   Fun for any kid past the toddler stage

★ ★ ★   Good for young hikers with proven stamina

★ ★   Not enjoyable for children

★   Not advisable for children

FOR DIFFICULTY:

★ ★ ★ ★ ★   Grueling

★ ★ ★ ★   Challenging, with stretches of ease

★ ★ ★   Moderate: won't beat you up—but you'll know you've been hiking

★ ★   Easy, with patches of moderate

★   Good for a relaxing stroll

FOR SOLITUDE:

★ ★ ★ ★ ★   Positively tranquil

★ ★ ★ ★   Spurts of isolation

★ ★ ★   Moderately secluded

★ ★   Crowded on weekends and holidays

★   Steady stream of individuals and/or groups

GPS TRAILHEAD COORDINATES

As noted in "Trail Maps," on page 3, I used a handheld GPS unit to obtain geographic data and sent the information to the publisher's cartographers. In the opener for each hike profile, the coordinates—the intersection of the latitude (north) and longitude (west)—will orient you at the trailhead. In some cases, you can drive within viewing distance of a trailhead. Other hikes require a short walk to reach the trailhead from a parking area. Either way, the trailhead coordinates are given from the trail's actual head—its point of origin.

This guidebook expresses GPS coordinates in degree–decimal minute format. For example, the coordinates for Hike 1, Raven Ridge Loop (page 20), are as follows: N39° 03.179' W79° 18.578'.

The latitude and longitude grid system is likely quite familiar to you, but here is a refresher, pertinent to visualizing the GPS coordinates.

Imaginary lines of latitude—called *parallels* and approximately 69 miles apart from each other—run horizontally around the globe. Each parallel is indicated by degrees from the equator (established to be 0°), up to 90°N at the North Pole and down to 90°S at the South Pole.

Imaginary lines of longitude—called *meridians*—run perpendicular to latitude lines. Longitude lines are likewise indicated by degrees starting from 0° at the Prime Meridian in Greenwich, England. They continue east and west until they meet 180° later at the International Date Line in the Pacific Ocean. At the equator, longitude lines also are approximately 69 miles apart, but that distance narrows as the meridians converge toward the North and South poles.

To convert GPS coordinates given in degrees, minutes, and seconds to degree–decimal minute format, divide the seconds by 60. For more on GPS technology, visit usgs.gov.

DISTANCE & CONFIGURATION

Distance notes the length of the hike round-trip, from start to finish. If the hike description includes options to shorten or extend the hike, those round-trip distances are also included here. **Configuration** defines the type of route—for example, a loop, an out-and-back (which takes you in and out the same way), a point-to-point (or one-way route), a figure-eight, or a balloon.

HIKING TIME

A general rule of thumb for the hiking times noted in this guidebook is 2 miles per hour. That pace typically allows time for taking photos, for dawdling and admiring views, and for alternating stretches of hills and descents. When deciding whether or not to follow a particular trail in this guidebook, consider the weather along with your own pace, general physical condition, and energy level on a given day.

HIGHLIGHTS

Lists outstanding features that draw hikers to the trail: mountain or forest views, water features, historical sites, and the like.

ELEVATION

Each hike's key information lists the elevation at the trailhead and other figures for the high and low points on the route. The full hike profile also includes a complete elevation profile (see page 4).

ACCESS

Trails in the Monongahela National Forest are open 24-7. Any applicable fees or permits required to hike the trail are listed here.

MAPS

Resources for maps, in addition to those in this guidebook, are listed here. As noted earlier, we recommend that you carry more than one map—and that you consult those maps before heading out on the trail.

FACILITIES

For planning your hike, it's helpful to know what to expect at the trailhead or nearby in terms of restrooms, water, picnic tables, and other niceties.

WHEELCHAIR ACCESS

Details the hike's feasibility for outdoor enthusiasts who use a wheelchair.

CONTACT

Listed here are ranger districts and their phone numbers for checking trail conditions, trail-access hours and seasons, and other day-to-day information before you head out. Also check the Monongahela National Forest website, fs.usda.gov/mnf, for information.

Overview, Route Details, Nearby Attractions, and Directions

These four elements compose the heart of the hike. **Overview** gives you a quick summary of what to expect on the trip. **Route Details** guides you on the hike, from start to finish. **Nearby Attractions** suggests appealing area sites, such as restaurants, museums, and other trails. **Directions** will get you to the trailhead from a well-known road or highway.

Weather

Each of the four seasons distinctly lay their hands on the Monongahela. Summer is generally mild—but humid—in the Allegheny Highlands. However, the lower parts of the national forest can—and will—have uncomfortable hot spells during the summer. Conversely, some of the highest terrain will be almost too cool in summer, especially during wet spells. Thunderstorms can pop up in the afternoons. Storm possibilities increase with elevation. Hikers get a little extra pop in their step when fall's first northerly fronts sweep cool, clear air across the Monongahela. Mountaintop vistas are best enjoyed during this time. Crisp mornings give way to warm afternoons. Fall is drier than summer and is the driest of all seasons. Winter can bring frigid subfreezing days and chilling rains—and copious snow in the high country. Elkins' annual snow average is 83 inches while White Sulphur Springs averages 17 inches. Marlinton gets 40 inches of the white stuff each year, while Bartow averages 67 inches. Obviously, adjacent highlands can receive much more. However, a brisk hiking pace will keep you warm. Each cold month will have a few days of mild weather. Nevertheless, be apprised that mild weather in the lowlands may still be frigid in the nearby highlands. Spring will be more variable. A warm day can be followed by a cold one. Extensive spring rains bring regrowth, but also keep hikers indoors. Moreover, spring rains can mean spring snow on the mountaintops. On average, March dumps the most inches of snow upon the region. Nevertheless, avid hikers will find more good hiking days than they will have time to hike in spring and every other season.

Water

How much is enough? A good rule of thumb is to hydrate prior to your hike, carry (and drink) 16 ounces of water for every mile you plan to hike, and hydrate again after the hike. For most people, the pleasures of hiking make carrying water a relatively minor price to pay to remain safe and healthy. So, pack more water than you anticipate needing, even for short hikes.

Water obtained in the backcountry presents inherent risks for thirsty trekkers. *Giardia* parasites contaminate many water sources and cause the dreaded intestinal giardiasis that can last for weeks after ingestion. For information, visit The Centers for Disease Control website at cdc.gov/parasites/giardia.

THE HIKE TO HIGH FALLS FIRST VISITS THE MEADOWS OF BEULAH. *(See Hike 22, page 114.)*

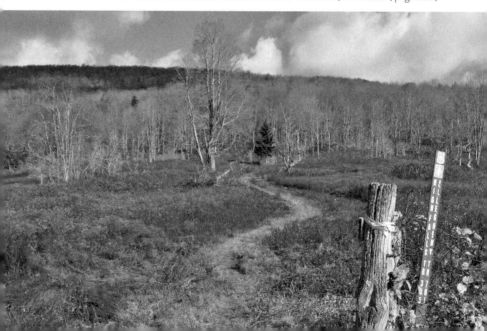

In any case, effective treatment is essential before using any water source found along the trail. Boiling water for two to three minutes is always a safe measure for camping, but day hikers can consider iodine tablets, approved chemical mixes, filtration units rated for *Giardia*, and UV filtration. Some of these methods (for example, filtration with an added carbon filter) remove bad tastes typical in stagnant water, while others add their own taste. Carry a means of purification to help in a pinch if you realize you have underestimated your consumption needs.

Clothing

Weather, unexpected trail conditions, fatigue, extended hiking duration, and wrong turns can individually or collectively turn a great outing into a very uncomfortable one at best—and a life-threatening one at worst. Thus, proper attire plays a key role in staying comfortable and, sometimes, in staying alive. Below are some helpful guidelines.

★ *Choose synthetics, silk, or wool* for maximum comfort in all of your hiking attire—from hats to socks and in between. Cotton is fine if the weather remains dry and stable, but you won't be happy if it gets wet.

★ *Always wear a hat,* or at least tuck one into your day pack or hitch it to your belt. Hats offer all-weather sun and wind protection as well as warmth if it turns cold.

★ *Be ready to layer up or down* as the day progresses and the mercury rises or falls. Today's outdoor wear makes layering easy, with such designs as jackets that convert to vests and zip-off legs.

★ *Wear hiking shoes or sturdy hiking sandals with toe protection.* Flip-flopping on a paved path in an urban botanical garden is one thing, but never hike mountain trails in open sandals or casual sneakers. The Monongahela can be very rocky. Your bones and arches need support, and your skin needs protection.

★ *Pair good footwear with good socks!* If you prefer not to sheathe your feet when wearing hiking sandals, tuck the socks into your day pack; you may need them if the weather plummets or if you hit rocky turf and pebbles begin to irritate your feet. And, in an emergency, if you have lost your gloves, you can wear the socks as mittens.

★ *Don't leave rainwear behind,* even if the day dawns clear and sunny. Tuck into your day pack, or tie around your waist, a jacket that is breathable and either water-resistant or waterproof. Investigate different choices at your local outdoor retailer. If you are a frequent hiker, ideally you'll have more than one rainwear weight, material, and style in your closet to protect you in all seasons in your regional climate and hiking microclimates.

Essential Gear

You can buy outdoor vests that have up to 20 pockets shaped and sized to carry everything from toothpicks to binoculars. Or, if you don't aspire to feel like a burro, you can neatly stow all of the following items (listed in alphabetical order, as all are important) in your day pack or backpack.

★ *Extra clothes:* raingear; a change of socks and shirt; and, depending on the season, a warm hat and gloves

★ *Extra food:* trail mix, granola bars, or other high-energy snacks

★ *Flashlight or headlamp* with extra bulb and batteries, for getting back to the trailhead if your hike takes longer than expected

★ *Insect repellent* to ward off ticks and other biting bugs

★ *Maps and a high-quality compass.* Even if you know the terrain from previous hikes, don't leave home without these tools. If you are versed with a GPS bring that, too, but don't rely on it as your sole navigational tool—batteries can die.

    The latest smartphones not only enable you to call for help but also have built-in GPS hardware and software that can help with orientation. However, don't call for help unless you truly need it, and remember that your phone's battery can die too. Smartphones are also valuable for downloading maps to use on the trail, although it's always better to download a map before your hike rather than trying to do so on the fly. Cell coverage in the Monongahela National Forest is very limited at best.

★ *Pocketknife and/or multitool*

★ *Sun protection:* sunglasses with UV tinting, a sunhat with a wide brim, and sunscreen. Be sure to check the expiration date on the tube or bottle.

★ *Water.* Bring more than you think you'll drink. Depending on your destination, you may want to bring a means of purifying water in case you run out.

★ *Whistle.* It could become your best friend in an emergency.

★ *Windproof matches and/or a lighter,* for real emergencies—please don't start a forest fire.

First Aid Kit

In addition to the items above, those below may appear overwhelming for a day hike. But any paramedic will tell you that the products listed here are just the basics. The reality of hiking is that you can be out for a week of backpacking and acquire only a mosquito bite—or you can hike for an hour, slip, and suffer a bleeding abrasion or broken bone. Fortunately, these items will collapse into a very small space. You may also purchase convenient, prepackaged kits at your pharmacy or online.

Consider your intended terrain and the number of hikers in your party before you exclude any article listed below. A short stroll may not inspire you to carry a complete kit, but anything beyond that warrants precaution. When hiking alone, you should always be prepared for a medical need. And if you're a twosome or a group, one or more people in your party should be equipped with first aid supplies.

★ Adhesive bandages (such as Band-Aids)

★ Antibiotic ointment (such as Neosporin)

★ Aspirin, acetaminophen (Tylenol), or ibuprofen (Advil)

★ Athletic tape

★ Blister kit (moleskin or an adhesive variety such as Spenco 2nd Skin)

★ Butterfly-closure bandages

★ Diphenhydramine (Benadryl), in case of mild allergic reactions

★ Elastic bandages (such as Ace) or joint wraps (such as Spenco)

★ Epinephrine in a prefilled syringe (EpiPen), typically by prescription only, for people known to have severe allergic reactions

★ Gauze (one roll and a half dozen 4-by-4-inch pads)

★ Hydrogen peroxide or iodine

General Safety

Here are a few tips to make your hike safer and easier:

★ *Always let someone know where you will be hiking and how long you expect to be gone.* It's a good idea to give that person a copy of your route, particularly if you are headed into an isolated area. Let them know when you return.

★ *Always sign in and out of any trail registers provided.* Don't hesitate to comment on the trail condition if space is provided; that's your opportunity to alert others to any problems you encounter.

★ *Don't count on a smartphone for your safety.* Reception will likely be nonexistent on the trail.

★ *Always carry food and water, even for a short hike.* And, again, bring more water than you think you'll need.

★ *Stay on designated trails.* Even on the most clearly marked trails, you usually reach a point where you have to stop and consider which direction to head. If you become disoriented, don't panic. As soon as you think you may be off track, stop, assess your current direction, and then retrace your steps to the point where you went astray. Using a map, a compass, a GPS device or smartphone, and this book, and keeping in mind what you have passed thus far, reorient yourself, and trust your judgment on which way to continue. If you become absolutely unsure of how to continue, return to your vehicle the way you came in. Should you become completely lost and have no idea how to return to the trailhead, remaining in place along the trail and waiting for help is most often the best option for adults and always the best option for children.

★ *Be especially careful when crossing streams.* Whether you are fording the stream or crossing on a log, make every step count. If you have any doubt about maintaining your balance on a log, ford the stream instead: use a trekking pole or stout stick for balance and face upstream as you cross. If a stream seems too deep to ford, turn back. Whatever is on the other side is not worth the risk.

★ *Be careful at overlooks.* While these areas may provide spectacular views, they are potentially hazardous. Stay back from the edge of outcrops, and make absolutely sure of your footing—a misstep can mean a nasty and possibly fatal fall.

★ *Standing dead trees and storm-damaged living trees pose a significant hazard to hikers.* These trees may have loose or broken limbs that could fall at any time. Look up while walking beneath trees and when choosing a spot to rest or enjoy a snack.

★ *Know the symptoms of subnormal body temperature, or hypothermia.* Shivering and forgetfulness are the two most common indicators of this stealthy killer. Hypothermia can occur at any elevation, even in the summer, especially if you're wearing lightweight cotton clothing. If symptoms develop, get to shelter, hot liquids, and dry clothes as soon as possible.

★ *Likewise, know the symptoms of heat exhaustion, or hyperthermia.* Here's how to recognize and handle three types of heat emergencies: Heat cramps are painful cramps in the legs and abdomen, accompanied by heavy sweating and feeling faint. Caused by excessive salt loss, heat cramps must be handled by getting to a cool place and sipping water or an electrolyte solution (such as Gatorade). Dizziness, headache, irregular pulse, disorientation, and nausea are all symptoms of heat exhaustion, which occurs as blood vessels dilate and attempt to move heat from the inner body to the skin. Find a cool place, drink cool water, and get someone to fan you, which can help cool you off more quickly. Heatstroke is a life-threatening condition that can cause convulsions, unconsciousness, or even death. Symptoms include dilated pupils; dry, hot, flushed skin; a rapid pulse; high fever; and abnormal breathing. If you should be sweating and you're not, that's the signature warning sign. If you or a hiking partner is experiencing heatstroke, do whatever you can to cool down and find help.

★ *Ask questions.* Monongahela National Forest employees are there to help. It is a lot easier to ask advice beforehand, and it will help you avoid a mishap away from civilization when it is too late to amend an error.

★ *Most important, take along your brain.* A cool, calculating mind is the single, most important asset on the trail. Think before you act. Watch your step. Plan ahead. Avoiding accidents before they happen is the best way to ensure a rewarding and relaxing hike.

Watchwords for Flora & Fauna

Black Bears

Though attacks by black bears are very rare, they have happened in the Appalachian Mountains. The sight or approach of a bear can give anyone a start. If you encounter a bear while hiking, remain calm and never run away. Make loud noises to scare off the bear and back away slowly. In primitive and remote areas, assume bears are present. In more-developed sites, check on the current bear situation prior to hiking. Most encounters are food related, as bears have an exceptional sense of smell and not particularly discriminating tastes. While this is of greater concern to backpackers and campers, on a day hike you may plan a lunchtime picnic or will munch on an energy bar or other snack from time to time. So remain aware and alert, especially at shelters along the Cranberry River, Allegheny Trail, and other popular national forest destinations.

Mosquitoes

These little naggers are more often found in urban areas but sparingly in the mountainous Monongahela, though they can be a nuisance in open agricultural valleys in the mountains. Insect repellent and/or repellent-impregnated clothing are the only simple methods to ward off these pests. In some areas, mosquitoes are known to carry the West Nile virus, so all due caution should be taken to avoid their bites.

Poison Ivy, Oak, and Sumac

Recognizing and avoiding poison ivy, oak, and sumac are the most effective ways to prevent the painful, itchy rashes associated with these plants. Poison ivy grows as a vine or groundcover, 3 leaflets to a leaf; poison oak grows as either a vine or shrub, also with 3 leaflets; and poison sumac flourishes in swampland, each leaf having 7–13 leaflets. Urushiol, the oil in the sap of these plants, is responsible for the rash. Within 14 hours of exposure, raised lines and/or blisters will appear on the affected area, accompanied by a terrible itch. Try to refrain from scratching because bacteria under your fingernails can cause an

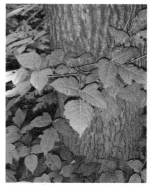

POISON IVY
Tom Watson

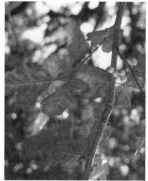

POISON OAK
Jane Huber

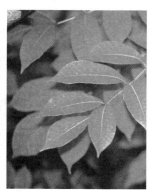

POISON SUMAC
Norman Tomalin/Alamy

infection. Wash and dry the affected area thoroughly with soap and water or a product such as Tecnu, then apply calamine lotion and/or an anti-itch cream. If itching or blistering is severe, seek medical attention. Likewise, make sure to wash any clothes, pets, or hiking gear that may have come in contact with the plant—you could experience a second breakout months after the first if you put on a shirt or a pair of boots that were never properly cleaned.

Snakes

Rattlesnakes, cottonmouths, copperheads, and coral snakes are among the most common venomous snakes in the United States, and hibernation season is typically from October through April. However, only two venomous snakes are native to West Virginia—the timber rattlesnake and the copperhead. The snakes you will most likely see while hiking will be nonvenomous species and subspecies. The best rule is to leave all snakes alone, give them a wide berth as you hike past, and make sure any hiking companions (including dogs) do the same.

When hiking, stick to well-used trails and wear over-the-ankle boots and loose-fitting long pants. Don't step or put your hands where you can't see, and avoid wandering around in the dark. Step *onto*

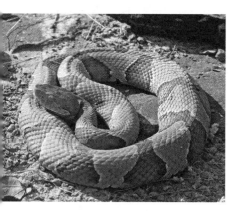

COPPERHEAD
Creeping Things/Shutterstock

logs and rocks, never *over* them, and be especially careful when climbing rocks. Always avoid walking through dense brush or willow thickets. Finally, don't peer into animal burrows, and make sure that dogs don't either.

Ticks

Generally speaking, tick encounters are rare in the Monongahela. Ticks are sometimes found on brush and tall grass, where they seem to be waiting to hitch a ride on a warm-blooded passerby. Adult ticks are most active April–May and again in October–November. The black-legged tick, or deer tick, is the primary carrier of Lyme disease. When hiking, wear light-colored clothing to make it easier to spot ticks before they make it to the skin. Afterward, visually check your hair, back of neck, armpits, and socks. During your posthike shower, take a moment to do a more complete body check. For ticks that are already embedded, removal with tweezers is best. Thoroughly clean the bite and your hands with disinfectant solution or soap and water. If you later feel ill or a red, ringlike rash develops around the bite, see a doctor.

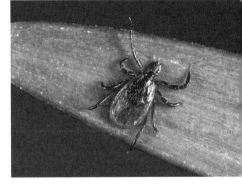

DEER TICK
Jim Gathany/Centers for Disease Control and Prevention (public domain)

Hunting

Separate rules, regulations, and licenses govern the various hunting types and related seasons in the Monongahela National Forest. Though there are generally no problems, cautious hikers may wish to forgo their trips during the big-game seasons, usually in November and December, when hunters are active. Consider wearing orange clothing or simply an orange vest and continuing with your plans.

Trail Etiquette

Always treat the trail, wildlife, and fellow hikers with respect. Respect the resource. Here are some reminders.

★ *Plan ahead in order to be self-sufficient at all times.* For example, carry necessary supplies for changes in weather or other conditions. A well-executed trip is a satisfaction to you and to others.

★ *Hike on open trails only.*

★ *Check conditions before you head out* if you think road or trail closures may be a possibility (use the websites or phone numbers listed in the "Contacts" section at the beginning of each hike profile). And don't try to circumvent such closures.

★ *Don't trespass on private land,* and obtain all permits and authorization as required. Leave gates as you found them or as directed by signage.

★ *Be courteous to other hikers, bikers, equestrians,* and others you encounter on the trails.

★ *Never spook wild animals or pets.* An unannounced approach, a sudden movement, or a loud noise startles most animals, and a surprised animal can be dangerous to you, to others, and to itself. Give them plenty of space.

★ *Observe any yield signs you encounter.* Typically, they advise hikers to yield to horses, and bikers to yield to both horses and hikers. A common courtesy on hills is that hikers and bikers yield to any uphill traffic. When encountering mounted riders or horsepackers, hikers can courteously step off the trail, on the downhill side if possible. Calmly greet riders before they reach you and don't dart behind trees. (You'll seem less spooky to the horse if it can see and hear you.) Also, don't pet a horse unless you're invited to do so.

★ *Practice Leave No Trace principles.* Leave the trail in the same shape you found it in, if not better. Also stay on the existing trail and don't blaze any new trails. Be sure to pack out what you pack in. No one likes to see the trash someone else has left behind. Visit lnt.org for more information.

Tips on Enjoying Hiking the Monongahela National Forest

Before you go, read the hike description in this book and visit the website for the Monongahela, though information is often limited. Call or visit the ranger station listed with each hike ahead of time if you have unanswered questions. This will help you get oriented to the forthcoming hike.

Investigate different destinations. The hikes within this guide traverse terrain varying over 3,700 feet in elevation while exploring ridges, streams, lakes, and geological and historical sights. Take a chance and make a new adventure instead of trying to recreate the same one over and over. You will be pleasantly surprised to see so many distinct landscapes in the Mon.

Take your time along the trails. Pace yourself. The landscapes along Monongahela National Forest trails are filled with wonders both big and small. Don't rush past a tiny salamander to get to that overlook. Stop and smell the wildflowers. Go ahead and take a seat on a trailside rock. Peer into a stream to find secretive fish. Take pictures. Make memories. Don't miss the trees for the forest.

We can't always schedule our free time when we want, but try to hike during the week and avoid the traditional holidays if possible. Trails that are packed in the summer are often clear during the colder months. Try to hike busy trails during off times. If you are hiking on a busy day, go early in the morning; it will enhance your chances of seeing wildlife.

THE MONONGAHELA PRESENTS MANY AQUATIC DESTINATIONS SUCH AS LICK BRANCH FALLS. *(See Hike 29, page 148.)*

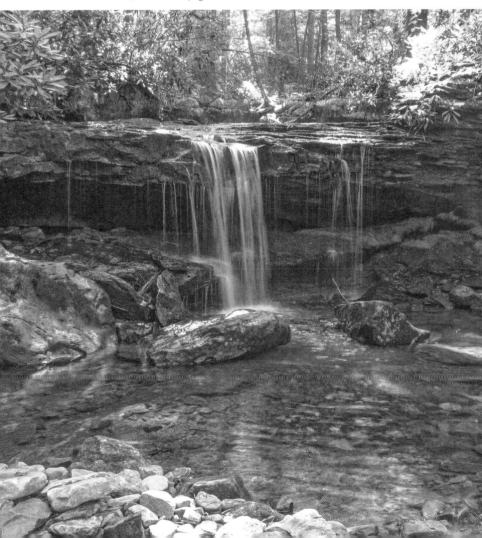

Dolly Sods Wilderness–Otter Creek Wilderness Area

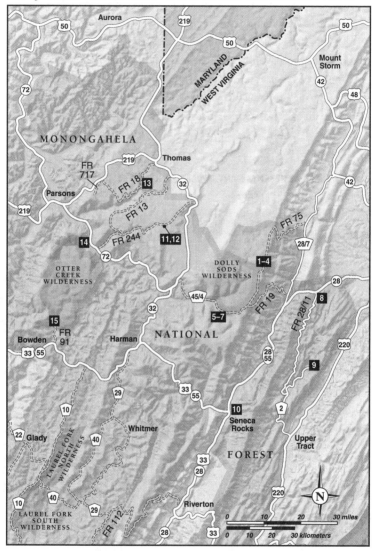

Dolly Sods Wilderness–
Otter Creek Wilderness Area

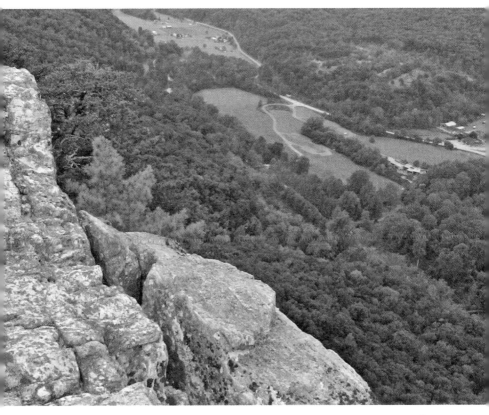

LOOKING DOWN ON THE DISCOVERY CENTER FROM SENECA ROCKS *(See Hike 10, page 59.)*

Raven Ridge Loop

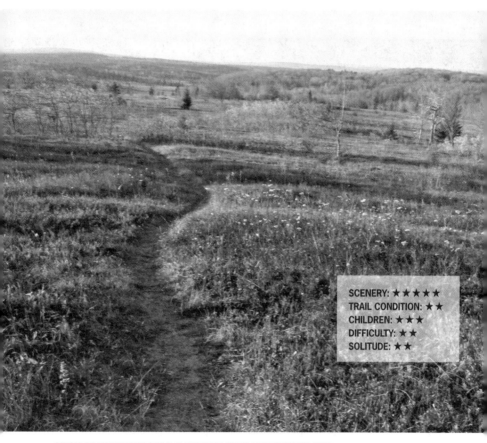

SCENERY: ★★★★★
TRAIL CONDITION: ★★
CHILDREN: ★★★
DIFFICULTY: ★★
SOLITUDE: ★★

MUCH OF THE DOLLY SODS PLATEAU IS OPEN TERRAIN LIKE THIS.

GPS TRAILHEAD COORDINATES: N39° 3.179' W79° 18.578'

DISTANCE & CONFIGURATION: 6-mile balloon

HIKING TIME: 3.5 hours

HIGHLIGHTS: Views galore, wilderness

ELEVATION: 4,080' at trailhead, 3,700' at low point

ACCESS: No fees or permits required

MAPS: *Dolly Sods Wilderness, Monongahela National Forest;* USGS *Blackbird Knob*

FACILITIES: Red Creek Campground with restrooms nearby

WHEELCHAIR ACCESS: None

CONTACT: Cheat-Potomac Ranger District, 304-257-4488

Overview

This circuit hike explores the north end of the Dolly Sods Wilderness, where meadows, heath glades, and grasses—all mixed with tree coppices—create an open landscape recalling the West. First, descend to Red Creek, gaining views from the first step. Come along the creek and head downstream in an open valley, where panoramas extend in all four cardinal directions. Turn up Raven Ridge, rising to more views. Cut through hardwoods and spruce, then reenter open vista-laden terrain. Cross Red Creek again, then descend a railroad grade in mixed woods and meadows before returning to the trailhead, amazed at the wealth of views.

Route Details

It is hard to watch your feet on this circuit hike because, most of the way, while traveling open lands with only scattered tree cover, you have views near and far. However, watch your feet you must, as segments of the hike pass through grassy wetlands, across mushy spring branches, and along sometimes-inundated logging grades. Moreover, there is one potential wet crossing of Red Creek. So take your time, enjoy the views of the north end of Dolly Sods Wilderness, and try not to get your feet wet—or just get 'em wet then don't worry about it.

Start your hike on the Beaver Dam Trail (a less-busy starting point than nearby Bear Rocks Trail), immediately dropping into the valley of upper Red Creek, backed by Cabin Mountain. Sparse forest cover allows you to see the hills and valleys of this perched plateau, with rock outcrops and spruce stands. Trace the path west through scattered and stunted tree coppices, along wet cranberry bogs, and through grasses.

At 0.7 mile, reach Dobbin Grade Trail. Turn left here, coursing down the open valley of Red Creek. As its name implies, the trail traces a former logging railroad grade that has a menagerie of grasses, stunted aspen, and rock gardens, but mostly open terrain. It won't be long before you reach your first wet section, often mushy grasses, or streamlets amid bogs, or just plain ol' mud holes. Try not to widen these wet spots by going far around them. Around you, the open terrain lends a different perspective on distance here in the mountains of West Virginia.

At 1.8 miles, come to the Red Creek crossing. Though the stream is small-ish here, expect to get your feet wet. Consider going barefoot but using trekking poles for balance, thus keeping your shoes and socks dry. Meet the Raven Ridge

Raven Ridge Loop

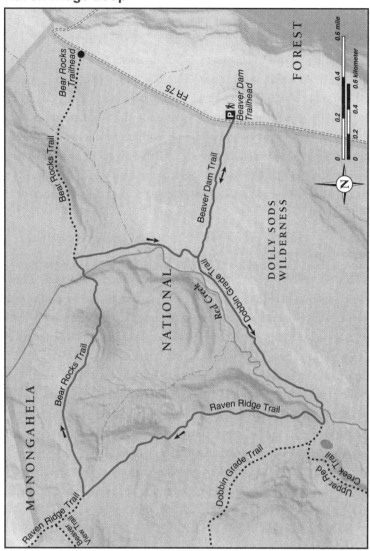

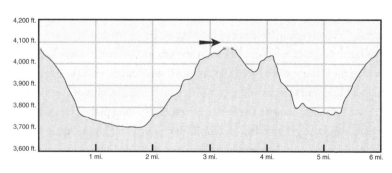

Trail shortly beyond the crossing. Turn right here, climbing the nose of a naked ridge cloaked in a few spruce and wind-flagged hardwoods. While climbing, look back for commanding panoramas of the lower Red Creek valley. Keep north as the balance of Dolly Sods Wilderness falls away to your south. This area deserves additional attention. Stop somewhere and just soak it all in.

At 2.6 miles, climb into woods then level off. Ahead, the trail winds through an ever-changing trailside of woods and meadows. Views still open to the west. Cabin Mountain forms a rampart and boundary of the Dolly Sods Wilderness. Bisect a spruce grove at 3.0 miles, then slice through a linear meadow ringed in spruce. At 3.3 miles in open terrain, meet the Bear Rocks Trail. Turn right on this path, now heading east in mostly open terrain. Look across the Dolly Sods and into the eastern horizon beyond the Allegheny Front, as well as far to the south of the Roaring Plains and even to the Seneca Creek Backcountry. What views!

Descend to reenter hardwoods at 4.1 miles. Cross several wetland boardwalks at 4.3 miles. Descend through hardwoods to rock-hop across Red Creek in a spruce thicket at 4.5 miles. Span one more boardwalk, then meet Dobbin Grade Trail at 4.6 miles. Turn right (south) here to experience an amalgam of meadow and forest, complete with mushy segments with Red Creek flowing roughly parallel to your right. The level grade lends itself to getting wet, since water runs slower on the flat surface that once carried timber from this howling back of beyond to market. Cross a little creek at 4.9 miles.

Meet the Beaver Dam Trail at 5.3 miles after making a sharp left and then a right. You have completed the loop portion of the hike. From here, it is 0.7 mile back to the Beaver Dam Trailhead, which you reach at 6.0 miles.

Nearby Attractions

Red Creek Campground, perched at nearly 4,000 feet, is one of the highest campgrounds in West Virginia. It is just a few miles south of the trailhead for this hike. The campground, open mid-April through November, offers 16 campsites in mixed woods and much open terrain. Each campsite has a picnic table, fire pit, and lantern post. It makes an ideal base camp for exploring the Dolly Sods Wilderness. Campground reservations are not available.

Directions

From Petersburg, drive west on WV 28 for 8.5 miles to County Road (CR) 28/7 (Jordan Run Road). Turn right on CR 28/7 and follow it 1.0 mile to Forest Road (FR) 19, on your left. Turn left on FR 19 and follow it 6.0 miles to FR 75. Turn right on FR 75 and follow it 6.5 miles to the Beaver Dam Trailhead, on your left.

A SPRUCE TREE RISES ABOVE THE DOLLY SODS.

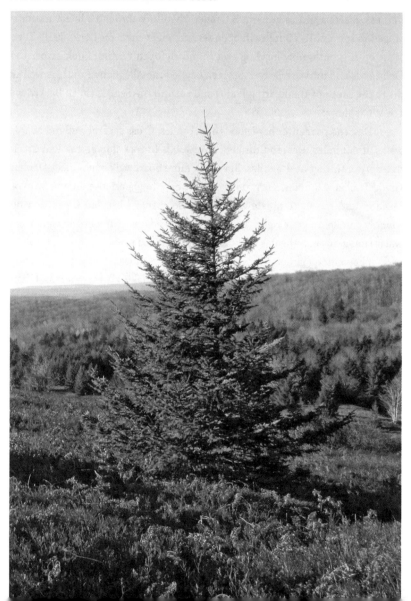

Blackbird Knob Vista

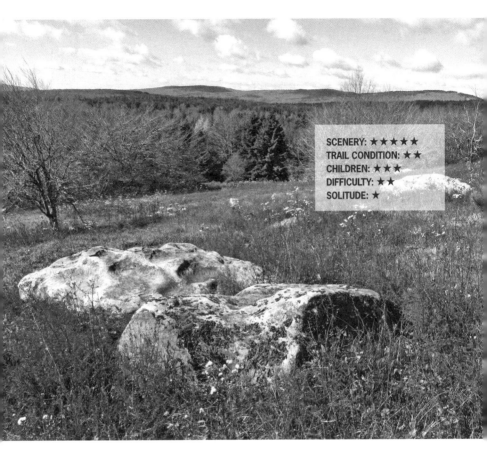

SCENERY: ★ ★ ★ ★ ★
TRAIL CONDITION: ★ ★
CHILDREN: ★ ★ ★
DIFFICULTY: ★ ★
SOLITUDE: ★

A VIEW INTO THE RED CREEK VALLEY FROM THE SOUTH SIDE OF BLACKBIRD KNOB

GPS TRAILHEAD COORDINATES: N39° 02.012' W79° 18.867'

DISTANCE & CONFIGURATION: 4.8-mile out-and-back

HIKING TIME: 2.5 hours

HIGHLIGHTS: Dolly Sods Wilderness, streams, views

ELEVATION: 3,900' at trailhead, 3,665' at low point, 3,980' at high point

ACCESS: No fees or permits required

MAPS: *Dolly Sods Wilderness, Monongahela National Forest;* USGS *Blackbird Knob*

FACILITIES: Red Creek Campground with restrooms nearby

WHEELCHAIR ACCESS: None

CONTACT: Cheat-Potomac Ranger District, 304-257-4488

Blackbird Knob Vista

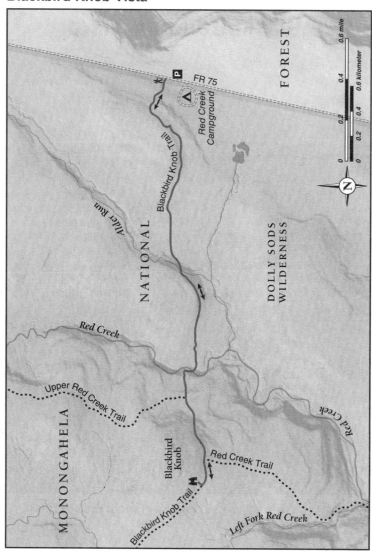

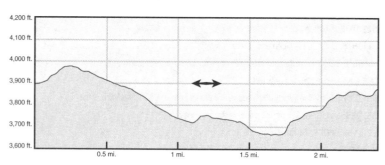

Overview

This hike explores a relatively newer portion of the Dolly Sods Wilderness, taking you to a secluded vista on the south side of Blackbird Knob. The Blackbird Knob Trail, which this hike uses, gives a good representation of the Dolly Sods, for this wealth of spruce forests, rock outcrops, clear streams, and open fields is a true treasure of the Monongahela. Elevation changes are insignificant, so you can concentrate on the views at hand rather than hanging your head and sucking wind. Do expect company on the hike, but not at the vista point.

Route Details

This is a special swath of the Monongahela National Forest. What is now the Dolly Sods Wilderness was a nearly impenetrable spruce forest. Then it was logged and burned over to bedrock. This left a landscape of heath meadows, rock outcrops, grasslands, and limited tree cover despite the work of the Civilian Conservation Corps, who planted trees in an effort to reforest the windswept land. During World War II, the Dolly Sods became a bombing target practice range and mountain maneuver area for the military. Later, its unique beauty was recognized and visitors began to trace its old logging roads and trails. The first portion of the Dolly Sods Wilderness was established in 1975. In 1997, munitions specialists came in and hunted shells in well-traveled areas. They found 15 shells and exploded them on-site. While the designated trails have been cleared of ordinance, it is still possible live shells or mortars are on site, so don't head off-trail. If you suspect you have found unexploded ordinance, don't touch or move it, then move away after recording where you found it and contact the U.S. Forest Service immediately. As a response to the obvious beauty and ongoing popularity of the Dolly Sods, it was expanded by more than 7,000 acres in 2009, raising it to 17,371 acres total.

This hike, which travels through the added wild area, is a good primer for experiencing Dolly Sods. Leave Forest Road (FR) 75 from the Blackbird Knob Trailhead. The Blackbird Knob Trail immediately leads you over a wetland on an elevated boardwalk. Begin climbing through a high-country woodland of yellow birch and maple stunted by the climate and flagged from winds. Alder thickets form along sluggish waters. This forest changes to spruce mixed with occasional open areas. Climb for 0.2 mile, then enter a planted grove of red pine, not native to the Dolly Sods.

Some muddy trail portions include stepping stones for dry-footed passage. At 0.4 mile, the trail opens onto a rocky area with great views to the southeast. To your left an open plain and forested ridge form a bowl around you. Continue to descend in a mostly open area, with cherry and aspen trees scattered about. Come to Alder Run at 1.1 miles, just downstream of a historically dammed beaver area. This is normally a simple rock-hop crossing.

From there, the Blackbird Knob Trail angles up a richly forested hillside, rising above bogs below. Skirt the south side of an unnamed knob. The trail stays rocky. Enter a cool and dark spruce forest just before coming to Red Creek at 1.7 miles. The trail seemingly ends on a small creekside bluff. Descend to the waters, then make a long rock-hop over the stream to a grassy area. Multiple campsites are in the vicinity. Parallel Red Creek upstream, then make a sharp left up a hill and away from the water.

Step into a wide plain, then meet the Upper Red Creek Trail at 1.9 miles. It leaves right for the northern part of the Dolly Sods Wilderness, but you stay west with the Blackbird Knob Trail. Enter an almost pure beech forest, yet another trailside ecotone. At 2.2 miles, come to a junction with the Red Creek Trail, which has come 6.4 miles from its other trailhead down by the Laneville Wildlife Cabin. Continue straight through this junction, entering a clearing at 2.3 miles. Uphill to your right is a boulder-pocked field. Climb off the Blackbird Knob Trail, leaving other hikers behind, and pick your favorite seat in the grandstand. Several outcrops amid the grasses beckon. The field is more level farther up. From your perch the gorge of Red Creek cuts a chasm below. Roaring Plains creates a wall to the south. The Allegheny Mountains rise on the horizon.

Nearby Attractions

Red Creek Campground, perched at nearly 4,000 feet, is one of the highest campgrounds in West Virginia, and is located within walking distance of the trailhead for this hike. The campground, open mid-April through November, offers 16 campsites in mixed woods and plenty of open terrain. Each campsite has a picnic table, fire ring, and lantern post. Campground reservations are not available.

Directions

From Petersburg, drive west on WV 28 for 8.5 miles to County Road (CR) 28/7 (Jordan Run Road). Turn right on CR 28/7 and follow it 1.0 mile to FR 19, on your left. Turn left on FR 19 and follow it 6.0 miles to FR 75. Turn right on FR 75 and follow it 5.0 miles to the Blackbird Knob Trailhead, on your left, just after passing Red Creek Campground.

Red Creek Falls via Fisher Spring Run

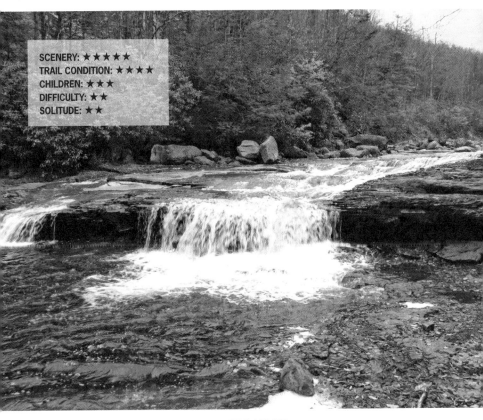

SCENERY: ★★★★★
TRAIL CONDITION: ★★★★
CHILDREN: ★★★
DIFFICULTY: ★★
SOLITUDE: ★★

LOWER RED CREEK FALLS SPILLS OVER LAYERED LEDGES.

GPS TRAILHEAD COORDINATES: N39° 0.403' W79° 19.649'

DISTANCE & CONFIGURATION: 4.8-mile out-and-back

HIKING TIME: 2.5 hours

HIGHLIGHTS: Cascades, Lower Red Creek Falls, Red Creek Falls

ELEVATION: 4,020' at trailhead, 3,040' at low point

ACCESS: No fees or permits required

MAPS: *Dolly Sods Wilderness, Monongahela National Forest;* USGS *Blackbird Knob, Hopeville*

FACILITIES: None

WHEELCHAIR ACCESS: None

CONTACT: Cheat-Potomac Ranger District, 304-257-4488

Red Creek Falls via Fisher Spring Run

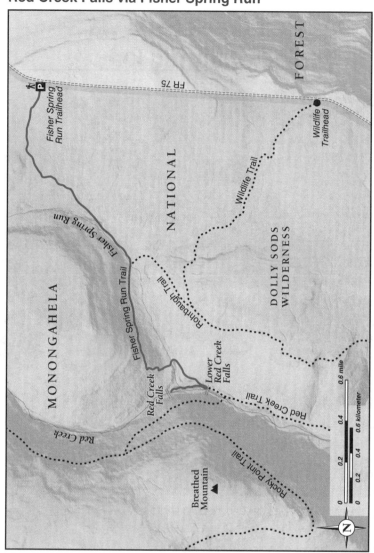

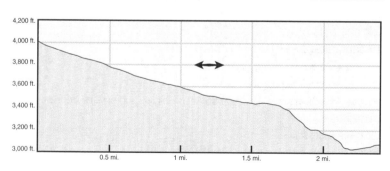

Overview

This hike ends with a lesser-visited reward—Red Creek Falls. Plus, your path to the falls takes a scenic route to get there. Start atop the Allegheny Front, then crisscross several small creeks before settling along an old railroad grade. Drop off the grade, then view cascades along Fisher Spring Run before reaching Red Creek. There, view wide Lower Red Creek Falls before making your way upstream to reach Red Creek Falls, a powerful rumbler with an immense pool. *Note:* The last 0.2 mile follows a fisherman's trail up to Red Creek Falls.

Route Details

Fisher Spring Run Trail is your conduit to view the falls on Red Creek located in the Dolly Sods Wilderness. It is one of the lesser-trod trails at Dolly Sods, despite being the shortest and best route to Red Creek Falls. In fact, because no trails go directly to Red Creek Falls, many hikers either pass it by or don't know about it at all. Trails pass near Lower Red Creek Falls, so, though it is less impressive than Red Creek Falls, it receives more visitation.

No need to fret over a little hiking on the unofficial trail at hike's end either. The walk up Red Creek from Lower Red Creek Falls to Red Creek Falls traces a nearly level fisherman's trail while passing through a few campsites. You then have to do a bit of rock-hopping (or simple wading) of Fisher Spring Run to reach Red Creek Falls. However, once there, you will be rewarded with a fine view of a 16-foot drop of aquatic force into a pool ideal for swimming in on a warm summer day.

Leave Forest Road (FR) 75, entering northern hardwoods and dropping off a hill on the Fisher Spring Run Trail. The singletrack path leads into a youngish forest, formerly fields. Such open terrain of the Dolly Sods is reforesting after a period of logging and sheep grazing. But not all of "The Sods"—as it is affectionately known—is grown over yet, as evidenced by a wet meadow you enter at 0.3 mile. Navigate a few more wet areas and several trickling branches that are ultimately feeding Fisher Spring Run.

By 0.9 mile, the trail comes alongside Fisher Spring Run, its tea-colored waters gurgling down a rocky bed. The path becomes rocky to the extreme and you enter a boulder field. Interestingly, at this juncture, Fisher Spring Run occasionally flows underground, leaving an often-dry bed, save for after storms and high water times.

However, this underground flow will be to your advantage. At 1.2 miles, intersect the Rohrbaugh Trail and its railroad grade. Turn right, joining the railroad grade as it crosses the extremely boulder-filled, but dry, bed of Fisher Spring Run. The railroad grade makes a gentle but steady descent into deep woods as Fisher Spring Run dives toward Red Creek at a greater decline.

At 1.7 miles, leave left from the railroad grade, descending a series of switchbacks on a declivitous and stony slope. Return to Fisher Spring Run at 1.9 miles. The creek emerges from the ground here in channels and is in the midst of a series of attractive cascades, none of which singly stand out, but the aggregate of them impresses. After this first crossing go left, upstream just a bit, then circle around a washout to cross another channel of the creek.

Pay close attention now. By 2.1 miles, you are now above Red Creek. A heavily used campsite lies below and you can hear Red Creek making some noise. Drop to the waterside campsite and work downstream just a bit to reach Lower Red Creek Falls. (If you intersect the Red Creek Trail you have gone too far.) Lower Red Creek Falls angles over a wide rock slab, drops about 8 feet over a ledge, then pushes downstream. Sunny ledges are abundant at this popular spot.

Now to Red Creek Falls. Keep upstream along Red Creek from Lower Red Creek Falls, passing through a few campsites in the woods. A fisherman's trail leads to the confluence with Fisher Spring Run, itself tumbling over boulders to finally meld into Red Creek. Rock-hop Fisher Spring Run, then work your way up along a partly vegetated gravel bar to reach Red Creek Falls. Here, Red Creek charges down a rockslide, then spills about 16 feet over an irregular rock ledge into a big, impressive pool. Waterside rock ledges create viewing platforms, though visitors will likely have to wet their feet for a complete and close-up examination of this waterfall, due to the depth and length of the pool below the falls.

Nearby Attractions

On the drive to this hike you will pass the Wildlife Trail parking area. The Wildlife Trail leads to the Rohrbaugh Overlook, one of the finest vistas in the entire Monongahela National Forest. That hike is also detailed in this guide on pages 33–36.

Directions

From Petersburg, drive west on WV 28 for 8.5 miles to County Road (CR) 28/7 (Jordan Run Road). Turn right on CR 28/7 and follow it 1.0 mile to FR 19, on your left. Turn left on FR 19 and follow it 6.0 miles to FR 75. Turn right on FR 75 and follow it 3.0 miles to the Fisher Spring Run Trailhead, on your left.

Rohrbaugh Overlook

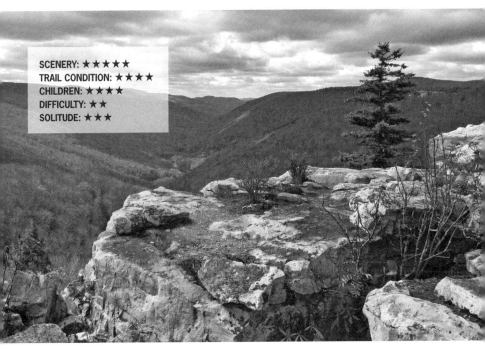

SCENERY: ★ ★ ★ ★ ★
TRAIL CONDITION: ★ ★ ★ ★
CHILDREN: ★ ★ ★ ★
DIFFICULTY: ★ ★
SOLITUDE: ★ ★ ★

THE OUTCROP AT ROHRBAUGH OVERLOOK STANDS ABOVE THE DEEP CUT OF
LOWER RED CREEK.

GPS TRAILHEAD COORDINATES: N38° 59.206' W79° 19.775'

DISTANCE & CONFIGURATION: 4.2-mile out-and-back

HIKING TIME: 2.5 hours

HIGHLIGHTS: Dolly Sods Wilderness, one of the best views in the entire national forest

ELEVATION: 4,020' at trailhead, 3,605' at low point

ACCESS: No fees or permits required

MAPS: *Dolly Sods Wilderness, Monongahela National Forest;* USGS *Hopeville*

FACILITIES: Red Creek Campground with restrooms nearby

WHEELCHAIR ACCESS: None

CONTACT: Cheat-Potomac Ranger District, 304-257-4488

Overview

This hike follows a former forest road down to the rim of the Red Creek Canyon.
From there it parallels the rim to an overlook at a huge outcrop availing views

Rohrbaugh Overlook

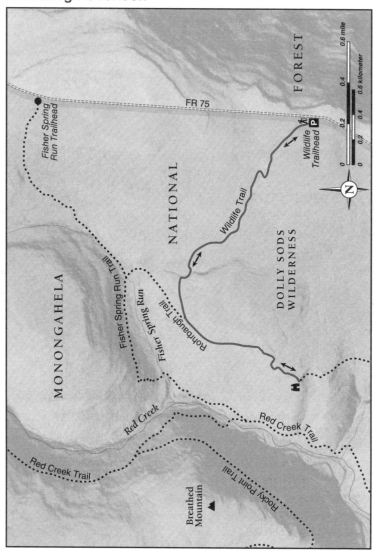

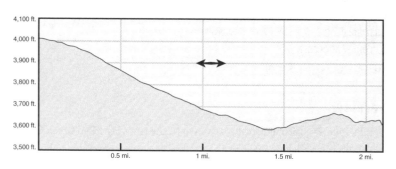

into the heart of the Dolly Sods Wilderness. The downgrade from the trailhead is moderate but steady. Along the way, you will pass relic meadows once managed for wildlife.

Route Details

Your route to Rohrbaugh Overlook—the Wildlife Trail—is so named because it was used by the U.S. Forest Service in pre-wilderness days to access and manage grassy food plots for game. These clearings can still be seen along the pathway. Though they are slowly growing over, the ecotones they create still contribute to the health of deer, bears, and turkeys that roam this part of the Monongahela National Forest.

Leave the trailhead, pass a trail signboard, then enter a deciduous forest of cherry, beech, and yellow birch, along with goosefoot maple. Immediately pick up the old forest road and descend, quickly passing the first former wildlife clearing on your left. The trailbed is partly grassy and is wet in places. The Dolly Sods Wilderness is known for having muddy trails. But there is a consolation here. The Wildlife Trail, since it follows a well-maintained former road, is largely devoid of boulders, so it is at least much less rocky than many other Dolly Sods trails.

Ease west down toward the Red Creek valley, making a wide switchback to the right at 0.4 mile. Step over a small stream. Make a sharp left turn at 0.5 mile, then parallel a streambed to your right. Pick your way through a rocky section at 0.9 mile, crossing stone-pocked intermittent streambeds. At 1.1 miles, step over a perennial stream banked against a hill. At 1.2 miles, the trail opens onto a big meadow. Grab a view of a knoll across the Fisher Spring Run valley. This big meadow was once sown with foods for wildlife, such as clover or corn. Since its wilderness designation in 1983, this meadow has been allowed to grow naturally. In the spots where the meadow is growing over, along its perimeter where field meets forest, are spots known as edges. These overlapping areas of ecotones are still rich food habitats despite the lack of U.S. Forest Service management, places where wild animals can find foods such as acorns from trees exposed to copious sunlight, wild fruits like blueberries and blackberries, and lush grasses. Eventually this former plot will give way to the northern hardwood forest and scattered evergreens that encircle it.

Stay along the left edge of the meadow, still descending. The Fisher Spring Run valley falls away to your right. At 1.4 miles, the Wildlife Trail ends. Keep straight, joining the Rohrbaugh Trail. To your right, the path drops off into Red

Creek. But follow the Rohrbaugh Trail straight, staying with the roadbed that will still prove to be easy on the feet compared to most other paths in the Dolly Sods.

The Rohrbaugh Trail turns south, working along the edge of the Red Creek Canyon dropping hundreds of feet below. The path is taking you below another formerly managed meadow. You will pass the acute left spur to access that meadow at 1.7 miles. At 1.8 miles, the old road splits. Staying left is the obvious choice, as the way to the right is growing over in trees. At 1.9 miles, bisect another meadow, coming to a perennial stream that you cross. Pass a couple of trails leading right to small outcrops with some views. These don't compare to what lies ahead. Reach a small clearing with more outcrops to your right.

Keep going. The trail becomes crowded by mountain laurel. At 2.1 miles, the path opens onto some massive, white rock cliffs on your right. There is no mistaking this area. Walk out here and take in the view. Below you and to the left is the lower Red Creek valley cutting a deep gorge, and even Red Creek itself is visible. The cliffs of Breathed Mountain stand out across the chasm. To the far left are more cliffs along the Rohrbaugh Trail, sometimes known as Lions Head Rock. To your right is the upper Red Creek valley. As you walk to the cliff's edge, note the distended outcrops accessible only by climbers, as well as diminutive mountain laurel, spruce, and other flora rising from small cracks in the rock. Look around and test the views from the varied stone protrusions—different outcrops produce different scenes. This is one of the best vistas in the entire Monongahela National Forest and a view worth every step of the way down—and back.

Nearby Attractions

Red Creek Campground, perched at nearly 4,000 feet, is one of the highest campgrounds in West Virginia and is located a few miles north of the trailhead for this hike. The campground, open mid-April through November, offers 16 campsites in mixed woods and much open terrain. Each campsite has a picnic table, fire ring, and lantern post. It makes an ideal base camp for exploring the Dolly Sods Wilderness. Campground reservations are not available.

Directions

From Petersburg, drive west on WV 28 for 8.5 miles to County Road (CR) 28/7 (Jordan Run Road). Turn right on CR 28/7 and follow it 1.0 mile to Forest Road (FR) 19, on your left. Turn left on FR 19 and follow it 6.0 miles to FR 75. Turn right on FR 75 and follow it 1.5 miles to the Wildlife Trailhead, on your left.

Dunkenbarger Loop

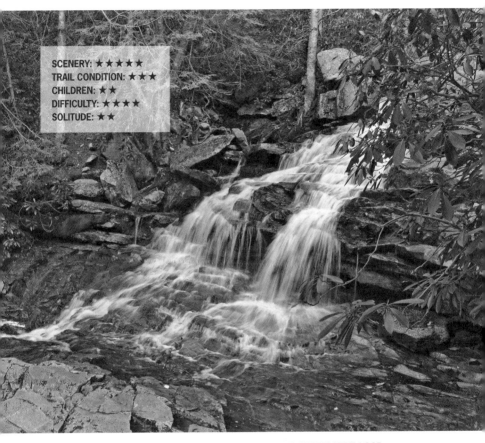

SCENERY: ★ ★ ★ ★ ★
TRAIL CONDITION: ★ ★ ★
CHILDREN: ★ ★
DIFFICULTY: ★ ★ ★ ★
SOLITUDE: ★ ★

BIG STONECOAL RUN FALLS IS BUT ONE HIGHLIGHT ON THIS SUPERLATIVE LOOP.

GPS TRAILHEAD COORDINATES: N38° 58.363' W79° 23.842'

DISTANCE & CONFIGURATION: 7.2-mile balloon

HIKING TIME: 3.5 hours

HIGHLIGHTS: Big Stonecoal Run Falls, varied ecosystems, wild streams

ELEVATION: 2,630' at trailhead, 3,730' at high point

ACCESS: No fees or permits required

MAPS: *Dolly Sods Wilderness, Monongahela National Forest*; USGS *Laneville, Hopeville*

FACILITIES: None

WHEELCHAIR ACCESS: None

CONTACT: Potomac Ranger District, 304-257-4488

Dunkenbarger Loop

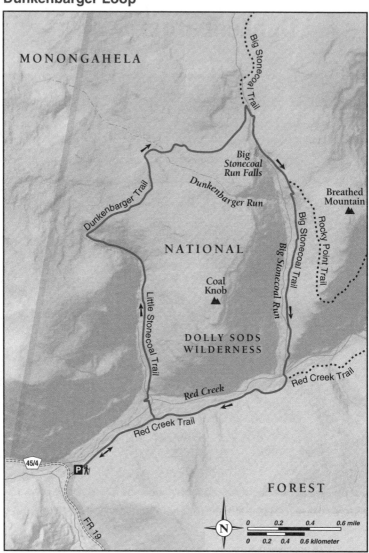

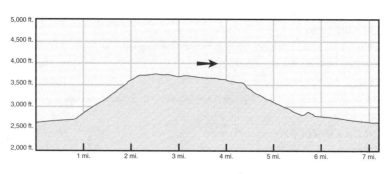

Overview

This hike traverses a lesser-visited area of the Dolly Sods Wilderness, due to a couple of fords. Start up Red Creek, then enter the deep valley of Little Stonecoal Run. Turn onto a high plateau via the Dunkenbarger Trail, traversing a scenic menagerie of spruce woods, meadows, and heath glades. Intersect Big Stonecoal Run, and descend past Big Stonecoal Run Falls while in this rugged valley. Return to Red Creek, finishing in a big, wild chasm. There are two crossings of Red Creek, which can be overly high in spring and after major rains. However, at normal water levels these crossing are very manageable.

Route Details

The solitude rating on this hike can be deceptive. You will likely see other hikers on Red Creek, but the first ford on this hike leaves most other trail trekkers behind. Depart the wooded parking area and head up the Red Creek Trail into the Dolly Sods Wilderness. Come directly alongside wide-bedded, rocky Red Creek at 0.3 mile. The valley of Little Stonecoal Run makes a cleft to your left, and the deep valley of Red Creek lies straight ahead. Leave the railroad grade you have been following and cross a feeder stream. Rock cairns help you navigate tricky areas. Beware user-created spur trails leading to campsites.

Reach a small meadow and signed trail junction at 0.6 mile. Turn left on the Little Stonecoal Trail (FT #552). Cruise through a wooded flat and reach Red Creek. Here is the crowd-thinning ford. Cross Red Creek just below the confluence with Little Stonecoal Run. Pick up the footpath, then hop over to the right bank of Little Stonecoal Run. You are now on a former logging road, shaded by oak, tulip, and black birch, making a steady ascent up the valley. At 1.5 miles, sneak past a low cliff line beside the trail, then look right for a small but dry rock house. At 1.7 miles, work your way past a slide.

The ascent takes you out of the oaks and into beech, yellow birch, and spruce trees. Rhododendron finds its place. Mosses cover boulders. Come to a red pine stand just before intersecting the Dunkenbarger Trail at 2.1 miles. The Little Stonecoal Trail just climbed nearly 800 feet in 1.3 miles.

Turn right on the Dunkenbarger Trail (FT #558) and ascend moderately around a knob. Soon level out in evergreen woods. At 2.5 miles, the forest canopy gives way to a heath glade of mountain laurel and blueberry bushes. Crowded spruce woods return later as you work through mucky sections. Hop

Dunkenbarger Run in a small clearing at 3.0 miles. This area is especially pretty, with grass, bushes, and trees all intermingled around the little stream.

Leave Dunkenbarger Run and keep heading east through a hodgepodge of spruce stands, heath glades, and small meadows. Work through a bog at 3.6 miles. Intersect the Big Stonecoal Trail at 3.8 miles. A large campsite stands near the intersection, shaded by spruce. Turn right on the Big Stonecoal Trail and soon rock-hop the dark, fast-moving Big Stonecoal Run to head downstream. Keep on a railroad grade as Big Stonecoal Run drops far off to your right.

Come to Big Stonecoal Run Falls at 4.0 miles, downhill to your right. A trail drops steeply to the worthy cataract. Here, Big Stonecoal Run drops about 20 feet, first in a widening arc, then briefly flattens out, and finally sprays downward a second time. Adjacent rock slabs make good observation spots.

Continuing down the trail, come along a stone cliff line before intersecting the Rocky Point Trail at 4.4 miles. It comes in on the railroad grade at you. Stay on Big Stonecoal Trail, and drop sharply right down a footpath. The stream is far below, but the noisy rapids echo through the sharp-sided valley. Keep dropping. The way is rocky and slow.

At 5.2 miles, work around a slide that has eroded the logging grade. Drop steeply as the valley widens before coming to Red Creek at 5.6 miles, where the trail seemingly ends at a flood-scoured bluff. Ease your way down to the water and cross the stream just above the confluence of Big Stonecoal Run and Red Creek. While in the open streambed of Red Creek, look left, upstream. The pale outcrops of the Rohrbaugh Overlook stand out at the head of the valley. Meet the Red Creek Trail just across the ford. Cut across the flat, then look for a path leaving the flat and switchbacking up the rocky hillside in front of you.

Ascend the hill, briefly pick up an old roadbed, and head downstream. Quickly leave the roadbed and follow a rocky, irregular path beneath maple and beech trees. Return to the valley floor, twice crossing a small branch. Meet the Little Stonecoal Trail at 6.6 miles. Retrace your steps down the Red Creek Trail back to the parking area, completing your loop at 7.2 miles.

Nearby Attractions

The Dolly Sods Wilderness is laced with 47 miles of trails to explore, and the adjacent Roaring Plains area has still more pathways to find.

Directions

From Petersburg, drive south on WV 28 for 8.5 miles to County Road (CR) 28/7 (Jordan Run Road). Turn right on CR 28/7 and follow it 1.0 mile to Forest Road (FR) 19, on your left. Turn left on FR 19 and follow it 6.0 miles to intersect FR 75. Here, turn left, staying with FR 19 , and drive 3.7 miles to the hamlet of Laneville. Look on your right for a brown building with a sign that says, LANEVILLE WILDLIFE CABIN. Turn right there and immediately come to the Red Creek Trail.

Alternate directions: From Harman, take WV 32 north 3.5 miles. Turn right on Bonner Mountain Road (CR 32/3). Follow CR 32/3 for 5.0 miles, then turn right on Laneville Road (CR 45/4). Follow CR 45/4 east 1.3 miles, crossing Red Creek on a road bridge. Immediately join FR 19 and turn left into the trailhead.

AN UPSTREAM VIEW OF RED CREEK

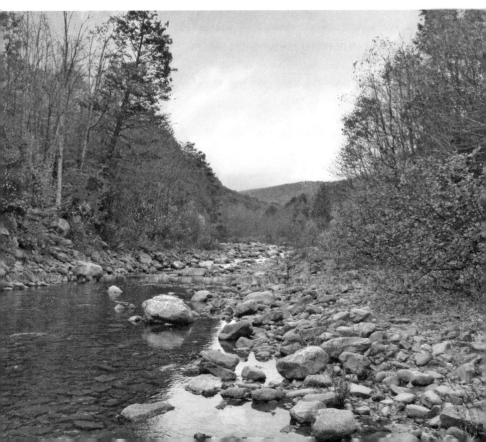

Boars Nest Loop

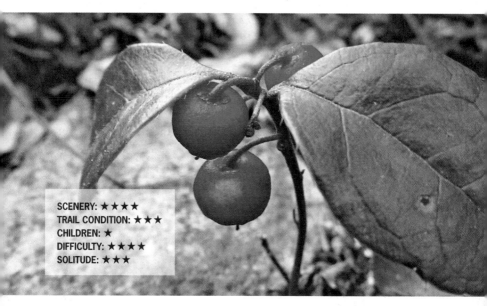

SCENERY: ★ ★ ★ ★
TRAIL CONDITION: ★ ★ ★
CHILDREN: ★
DIFFICULTY: ★ ★ ★ ★
SOLITUDE: ★ ★ ★

CRANBERRIES CAN BE FOUND IN SOME OF THE TRAILSIDE HEATH GLADES.

GPS TRAILHEAD COORDINATES: N38° 57.679' W79° 23.356'

DISTANCE & CONFIGURATION: 7.1-mile loop

HIKING TIME: 4 hours

HIGHLIGHTS: Heath glades, streams, views

ELEVATION: 2,990' at trailhead, 2,815' at low point, 4,290' at high point

ACCESS: No fees or permits required

MAPS: *Roaring Plains West, Monongahela National Forest;* USGS *Hopeville*

FACILITIES: Red Creek Campground with restrooms nearby

WHEELCHAIR ACCESS: None

CONTACT: Cheat-Potomac Ranger District, 304-257-4488

Overview

This hike loops through the Flatrock–Roaring Plains area, squeezed between Dolly Sods Wilderness to the north and Roaring Plains West Wilderness to the west. This area is much like the adjacent wildernesses, but it receives fewer visitors. Climb the scenic South Fork Red Creek valley, then do a little walking on a gated forest road. Turn onto the Boars Nest Trail, meeting the magnificent Flatrock Plains, mantled in a sightly spruce and heath forest. Before you leave the plains, grab a great view of the Dolly Sods to your north. Finally, drop steeply back down to South Fork. This very sharp descent accounts for much of the difficulty rating for this hike.

Route Details

This hike does have two creek crossings that might be troublesome in high water. Start your climb on the gated forest road leaving the parking area. Join the South Prong Trail, descending toward South Fork Red Creek. This is the lower trailhead of South Prong Trail, and it traces old Forest Road (FR) 479. Make a gentle walk 0.6 mile down to boulder-strewn South Fork. Rock-hop South Fork and turn left, tracing the watercourse upstream. Do not turn right to follow old FR 479 after crossing.

Soon, turn away from South Fork, climbing alongside a small stream to your right. Turn back up the main valley, picking up a logging grade at 1.0 mile under hardwoods mixed with mossy boulders. Follow the grade left for 0.2 mile, then follow the split right, uphill, to pick up a second logging grade at 1.5 miles. This may seem confusing, but the trail is clearly marked.

Stay with this grade as it gently ascends the South Fork valley. Cross occasional wet areas. Rhododendron groves pop up. Curve south into the upper South Prong valley. Red spruce begins to make a presence. At 2.6 miles, come across metal relics from what seems to be an old logging camp on your right. Just beyond here, drop left and cross the dark-colored South Fork. Resume climbing, enclosed by rhododendron. At 3.1 miles, leave the grade and clamber steeply to your right a short distance to seasonally closed FR 70. This road is primarily used to maintain a gas pipeline on leased national forest land. Turn right on FR 70, heading southwest. The roadside forest becomes predominately spruce.

At 4.5 miles, pass a rough road leaving left. Just past this side road, on your right, is the signed Boars Nest Trail. Turn onto the Boars Nest Trail and enter woods, reaching and crossing the headwaters of South Fork Red Creek. Spruce, moss, and rocks reign here. Climb out of the watershed and onto the Flatrock Plains at 4.9 miles. Low-lying shrubs such as mountain laurel, cranberry, and blueberry are punctuated with spruce trees, whose tops flag to the east, a reflection of the harsh and regular winds that fall upon this area, especially in winter.

Enjoy this beautiful stretch of trail on a stone-lined pathway that keeps you out of wet areas where cranberries grow. The canopy closes briefly. The forest, rife with mountain ash here, opens back up, and fine views spread out

Boars Nest Loop

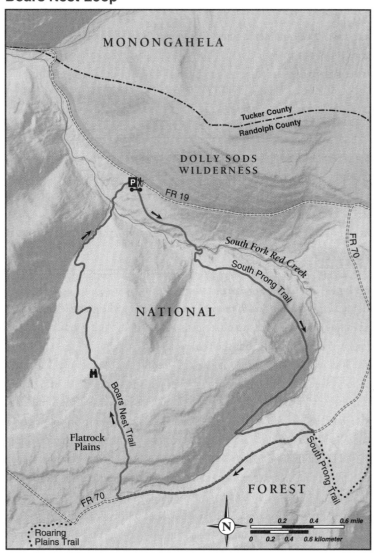

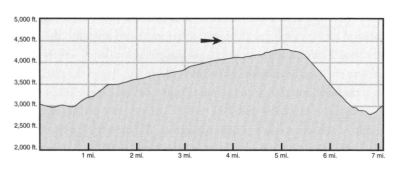

before you. The Dolly Sods stand dead ahead to your north. There is an outcrop to your left at mile 5.4, which makes a superlative resting and viewing location. It is a long way down from here.

Begin to drop off the Flatrock Plains, but soak in a few more views before you penetrate the tree canopy for good. Pass a spring branch and plunge downward through yellow birch woodland. Keep the brakes on this declivitous stretch. Make a pair of switchbacks at mile 5.9.

Keep descending. An unnamed tributary of South Fork, flowing off the Flatrock Plains, becomes plainly audible and visible to your left. Come along the side stream, then make another bridgeless crossing of South Fork at 6.9 miles. Congratulations, you just descended 1,400 feet in 1.3 miles. Woe to the hiker going in the other direction.

Leave the creekbed and climb uphill through a rocky oak and maple forest. Intersect two old woods roads before coming to the trailhead parking area, completing your loop at 7.1 miles.

Nearby Attractions

Red Creek Campground, perched at nearly 4,000 feet, is one of the highest campgrounds in West Virginia, and is located about 5 miles north of the trailhead for this hike. The campground, open mid-April through November, offers 16 campsites in mixed woods and much open terrain. Each campsite has a picnic table, fire ring, and lantern post. It makes an ideal base camp for exploring the Dolly Sods Wilderness. Campground reservations are not available.

Directions

From Petersburg, drive south on WV 28 for 8.5 miles to County Road (CR) 28/7 (Jordan Run Road). Turn right on CR 28/7 and follow it 1.0 mile to FR 19, on your left. Turn left on FR 19 and follow it 6.0 miles to intersect FR 75. Here, turn left, staying with FR 19 and follow it 2.7 miles to the Boars Nest–South Prong Trailhead. On the way you will pass the upper South Prong Trailhead. Start your hike at the lower South Prong Trailhead.

Alternate directions: From Harman, take WV 32 north for 3.5 miles to turn right on Bonner Mountain Road (CR 32/3). Follow CR 32/3 for 5.0 miles, then turn right on Laneville Road (CR 45/4). Follow Laneville Road east 1.3 miles, crossing Red Creek on a road bridge. Immediately join FR 19. Pass the lower Red Creek Trailhead and stay on FR 19 for 1.1 more miles. Turn right into the trailhead.

Red Creek Plains

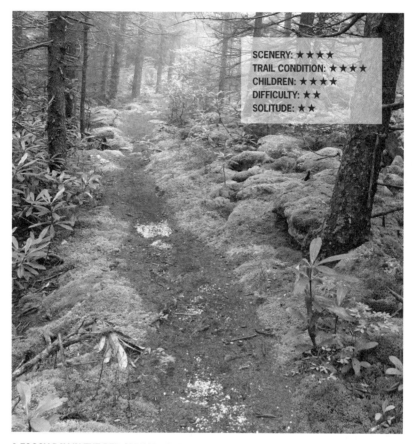

A FOGGY DAY IN THE RED SPRUCE FOREST OF THE RED CREEK PLAINS

SCENERY: ★ ★ ★ ★
TRAIL CONDITION: ★ ★ ★ ★
CHILDREN: ★ ★ ★ ★
DIFFICULTY: ★ ★
SOLITUDE: ★ ★

GPS TRAILHEAD COORDINATES: N38° 57.508' W79° 21.571'

DISTANCE & CONFIGURATION: 3.4-mile out-and-back

HIKING TIME: 2.5 hours

HIGHLIGHTS: Boardwalks, high elevation, views, wetlands

ELEVATION: 3,920' at trailhead, 4,085' at high point

ACCESS: No fees or permits required

MAPS: *Roaring Plains West, Monongahela National Forest;* USGS *Petersburg West, Hopeville*

FACILITIES: None

WHEELCHAIR ACCESS: None

CONTACT: Cheat-Potomac Ranger District, 304-257-4488

Overview

This is an excellent all-ages hike for those who want a taste of the Roaring Plains area adjacent to Dolly Sods. Explore high-elevation bogs, and get a view as a reward at the end. Elevation changes are less than 200 feet. Take the South Prong Trail through wetlands, keeping your feet dry by taking 12 boardwalks through the fragile areas. Alternately ramble through dense spruce forests, heath glades, and rock gardens. A short final ascent takes you to a knob where a short spur leads to a rocky clearing with a vista.

Route Details

This hike traverses the Red Creek Plains, a mostly forested area of high-altitude wetlands, rock outcrops, and spruce forests. The trail over the plains—South Prong—is fairly level, making a rewarding trek for hikers of all ages, especially those wary of trekking deep into the greater Dolly Sods–Roaring Plains area.

Once, this area was completely forested. Following logging, wildfires burned what was left of the woods down to bedrock. The relatively level ridge top and lack of vegetation lent a plain-like look to the place, giving the Red Creek Plains a name that fits less and less each passing year. It has taken several decades for the vegetation to return, including not only red spruce but also the heath glades and wetlands. Despite the rising spruce, excellent views still remain, as well as attractive environments such as open bogs of moss and tundra flora, including wild cranberries. Look also for heath glades, which are low-lying plant communities of mountain laurel, azalea, and blueberry. Legend has it that back in the Great Depression of the 1930s, the Red Creek Plains were repeatedly burned in order to foster wild blueberry growth. The berries were then eaten by hungry locals. The original logging of the area took place between the 1880s and the 1920s. Soil-stripping wildfires followed the logging, and the aforementioned blueberry-stimulating fires played a part in the slow return of the forest.

Start your hike on the upper South Prong Trail. Head south along a high, flat ridge that forms part of the Allegheny Front—the point where streams east and west of this plateau flow directly into the Atlantic Ocean via the Potomac River watershed on the east and from Red Creek, then river to river, and eventually to the Gulf of Mexico on the west.

Quickly join a boardwalk that crosses and preserves a wet bog below you. This is the first of 12 such boardwalks that are installed on the first 0.8 mile of path. These boardwalks extend from 10 feet to more than 100 feet in length. The

Red Creek Plains

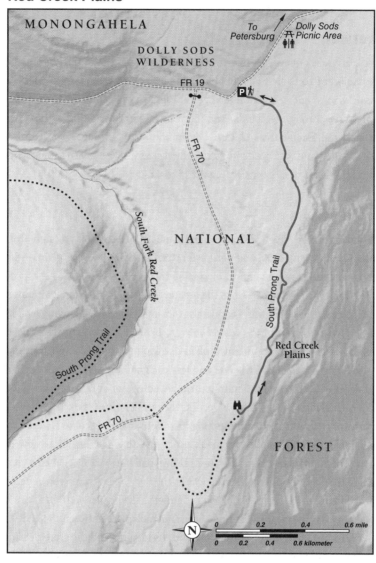

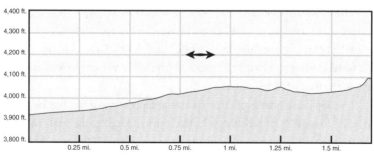

raised bridges allow water to pass naturally under you instead of being dammed by a grooved trail. Much of this initial section is also graveled, making for easier passage and better drainage. After rainy periods, the trailbed can still be wet.

Between the numerous wet clearings are stands of spruce and small meadows. The canopy is open overhead more often than not. The trail can be rocky, and the dense vegetation lends an almost claustrophobic character to the trail, despite often being open overhead. Off-trail hiking is discouraged here. Not only is it extremely difficult, but the sensitive vegetation cannot stand too much stomping.

Pass through a boulder field at 0.7 mile. Beyond the boulder field, the vegetation closes in again. At 1.0 mile, the South Prong Trail makes a sharp turn to the right and then eventually resumes its southbound ways. Top out on a rock flat, strewn with boulders, at 1.1 miles. You are encircled by spruce. Look for partial views of the wooded Flatrock Plains and South Fork Red Creek valley to your west.

At 1.2 miles, descend between some large, dark boulders into a thick spruce wood. A faint spur heads to a rock outcrop with more views. The trail continues to alternate environments rapidly—spruce groves, heath glades, rock gardens, and laurel thickets. The locale even includes some northern red oak trees. They grow low and wide in response to the harsh conditions.

At 1.6 miles, make the only significant climb of the hike. And this one is short. Once you top out, look for a slender trail leading to your right. Walk about 50 feet to a talus slope. This is your Red Plains grandstand. Here, views open up to your north and east. South Fork Red Creek is below you. The Dolly Sods lie in the northern distance. To your east are the mountains beyond the Allegheny Front. See if you can find regenerating American chestnut around here. They add an exclamation point to the vegetation variety—and views—found on this hike.

Nearby Attractions

Along the way to the trailhead you will pass the Dolly Sods Picnic Area, with shaded tables and a restroom.

Directions

From Petersburg, drive west on WV 28 for 8.5 miles to County Road (CR) 28/7 (Jordan Run Road). Turn right on CR 28/7 and follow it 1.0 mile to Forest Road (FR) 19, on your left. Turn left on FR 19 and follow it 6.0 miles to meet FR 75. Stay left on FR 19 and follow it 1.0 mile more to the upper South Prong Trailhead on your left a little after the Dolly Sods Picnic Area.

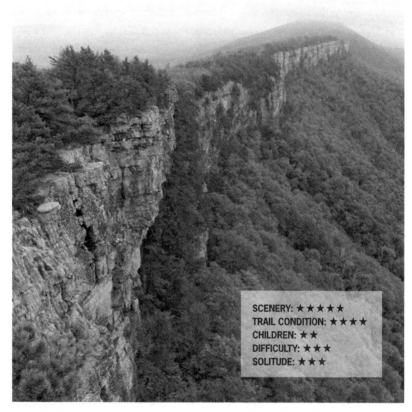

8 Chimney Top

SCENERY: ★★★★★
TRAIL CONDITION: ★★★★
CHILDREN: ★★
DIFFICULTY: ★★★
SOLITUDE: ★★★

THIS VIEW ALONG NORTH FORK MOUNTAIN DEFINES THE BEAUTY OF THE
MONONGAHELA NATIONAL FOREST.

GPS TRAILHEAD COORDINATES: N38° 58.884' W79° 13.872'

DISTANCE & CONFIGURATION: 5-mile out-and-back

HIKING TIME: 2.5–3 hours

HIGHLIGHTS: Chimney Top, extensive views, falcons, geology

ELEVATION: 1,120' at trailhead, 3,080' at high point

ACCESS: No fees or permits required

MAPS: *North Fork Mountain Trail, Monongahela National Forest;* USGS *Petersburg West, Hopeville*

FACILITIES: None

WHEELCHAIR ACCESS: None

CONTACT: Cheat-Potomac Ranger District, 304-257-4488

Overview

This is one of the best day hikes not only in the Monongahela National Forest but also in the whole of West Virginia. The entire walk is interesting—and challenging. First, pass an old homesite, and while on your way to great views, maybe you'll be lucky enough to see a peregrine falcon. They nest on the rocky west side of North Fork Mountain. Excellent views are a sure reward. However, you have to climb to get there, gaining almost 2,000 feet on the way. Bring water; there is none on the trail.

Route Details

North Fork Mountain is one of the Monongahela National Forest's special places. It is a north–south running ridge separating the South Branch Potomac River from the North Fork of the South Branch Potomac River. Serrated with gray sandstone outcrops running along its crest, North Fork Mountain recalls the Chimney Rocks, as well as other outcrops such as the Champe Rocks and the world-famous Seneca Rocks. The sheer cliffs, knobs, and ragged upthrusts of North Fork Mountain attract hikers and climbers. Yet other parts of the mountain are cloaked in craggy pines, laurel thickets, and even wild azalea stands. Most common are hickory-oak woods. Peregrine falcons have historically nested on North Fork Mountain and do to this day. Golden eagles are also known to swoop among the mountain's elevations. Kile Knob, at 4,588 feet, is the mountain's high point.

Our hike to Chimney Top starts much lower and, despite ascending nearly 2,000 feet, barely breaks the 3,000-foot marker. Start on the singletrack North Fork Mountain Trail off Smoke Hole Road. Immediately climb a small hill, then pass an old homesite on your left. The level area is growing up in forest. Notice the rock piles on the nearby hillsides; this indicates once-tilled or pasture land. Briefly connect to an old woods road heading back to the homesite, then begin a steady rise through pine-hickory-oak woodland growing over the rocky soil.

At 0.5 mile, the trail swings left onto a piney point of a ridge. Mountain laurel and blueberry grow in abundance beneath the conifers and black gum trees. Enjoy the level stretch, then climb around the heads of some dry coves before coming to another point of a ridge at 0.8 mile. Additional switchbacks take you up the side of North Fork Mountain. Obscured views extend north of Petersburg but don't compare to the vistas ahead. Make an abrupt right turn at 1.3 miles.

Come to your first outcrop at 1.7 miles. This is the beginning of the escarpment that runs along the west side of the mountain. Look to your left and you can

Chimney Top

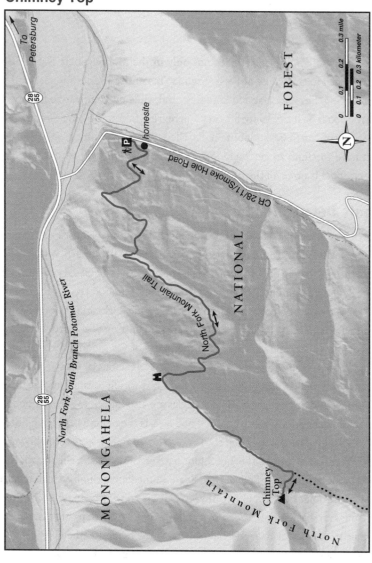

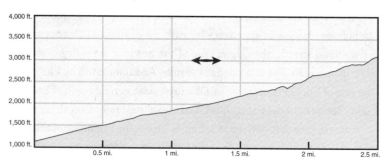

see the wall of stone rising up the mountain. Admire the abundance of Virginia pine atop the ridge here. Below, WV 28/55 runs alongside the North Fork of the South Branch Potomac River as it cuts a water gap between North Fork Mountain and New Creek Mountain. Down on the highway, you can see the entrance building of Smoke Hole Caverns, a privately operated cave, among other structures.

Make a southern track along the ridge, paralleling the escarpment. Grand vistas lie to your right just a few steps away. User-created trails extend to the crest and more of those irresistible panoramas. At 2.2 miles, the ridge rises well above the trail. Begin to look for a pile of white rocks that mark the spur leading right to Chimney Top. At 2.4 miles, the side trail to Chimney Top heads straight up the ridge through black gum, mountain laurel, pines, and chestnut oaks.

Follow this user-created spur. Continue around 200 feet up to the nearly continual rock outcrop atop the ridge. The actual Chimney Rock is the highest one you see. It takes a little climbing. Be careful, there is sand on the rocks here. A USGS survey marker lies atop the rock at 2.5 miles. What a view! From here, you can look south along the long escarpment and the balance of North Fork Mountain fading in the distance. Below flows the North Fork. To the west rises the high plateau of Dolly Sods. Keep your eye on the sky for falcons, eagles, and vultures riding the thermals around you. The multiple rock outcrops and vantages will keep you hopping around Chimney Top. Just be careful and take your time soaking in the first-rate West Virginia mountain scenery here in the Monongahela National Forest.

Nearby Attractions

North Fork Mountain Trail extends from this trailhead along the rocky length of North Fork Mountain for a total of 24 miles, making for a scenic yet dry hike (bring water). Views are numerous, but the path can be steep, even on the crest. Its southern terminus is on private property and not recommended. However, in addition to this hike, the North Fork Mountain Trail can be accessed by the Landis Trail as well as the Redman Run Trail. They both start off of Smoke Hole Road.

Directions

From Petersburg, drive 6.0 miles west on WV 28 to County Road (CR) 28/11 (Smoke Hole Road). Look for the sign for Smoke Hole Recreation Area and Big Bend Campground. Turn left to immediately cross the North Fork of the South Branch Potomac River, then continue up CR 28/11 for 0.3 mile. The signed North Fork Mountain Trail will be on your right.

Big Bend Loop

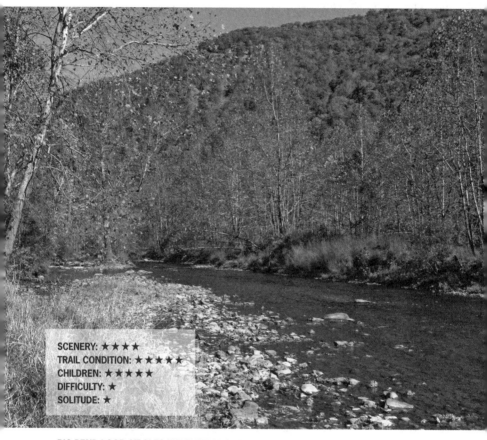

SCENERY: ★★★★
TRAIL CONDITION: ★★★★★
CHILDREN: ★★★★★
DIFFICULTY: ★
SOLITUDE: ★

BIG BEND LOOP CIRCLES THROUGH SMOKE HOLE CANYON.

GPS TRAILHEAD COORDINATES: N38° 53.482' W79° 14.450'

DISTANCE & CONFIGURATION: 1.2-mile loop

HIKING TIME: 1 hour

HIGHLIGHTS: Bluffs, camping, South Branch Potomac River

ELEVATION: 1,195' at trailhead, 1,275' at high point

ACCESS: No fees or permits required

MAPS: *Monongahela National Forest;* USGS *Hopeville*

FACILITIES: Restrooms, water, campground in season

WHEELCHAIR ACCESS: None

CONTACT: Cheat-Potomac Ranger District, 304-257-4488

Overview

This circuit hike is set in the Smoke Hole Canyon of the South Branch Potomac River. Here, the trail makes a loop, following Big Bend as the river nearly doubles back on itself. You leave the day-use area and climb a knob, coming to the neck of the Big Bend. From there, trace the clear river as it flows downstream around Big Bend Campground. Pass the chimney of a post office from days gone by before returning to the trailhead. Since this is a short hike, consider combining your walk with swimming, fishing, tubing, or camping.

Route Details

Big Bend lies in a dramatic setting, perched on a teardrop-shaped peninsula, with the South Branch Potomac River nearly encircling the area. On the outside of the river, wooded cliffs rise to form a natural cathedral. Old-timers called this the Smoke Hole because the mist rising from the deep gorge reminded them of smoke emerging from a cavity in the ground.

Nearly everyone can enjoy the Big Bend Trail. It is not too steep, not too long, and delivers eye-pleasing scenery every step of the way while circling the peninsula and adding a little history. Moreover, if anyone in your party is not crazy about hiking, you can entice them with additional activities such as picnicking, camping, fishing, swimming, paddling, or tubing.

As you enter the day-use area, join the Big Bend Trail leaving right, just before the Big Bend Campground gate. The singletrack hiking trail angles up a hill. A few switchbacks mitigate the climb. Oak, pawpaw, hickory, sassafras, and maple shade the trail.

Climb onto a ridgetop and reach the high point of the hike at 0.2 mile. The ascent is less than 100 feet. Here, trails go left and right. The left trail goes to the Upper Loop of Big Bend Campground. The Upper Loop is actually two loops. The sites up there do not have tent pads, but there are water spigots everywhere and a nice bathhouse for your convenience. White pine and autumn olive grow in great abundance here.

The Big Bend Trail heads right, away from the Upper Loop, descending on a rock-lined path to soon meet a spur trail leading right to alternate parking at the neck of the Big Bend peninsula. Stay with the Big Bend Trail as it works its way downstream along a rocky, piney hillside with outcrops and bluffs. Spur trails lead toward the river.

Big Bend Loop

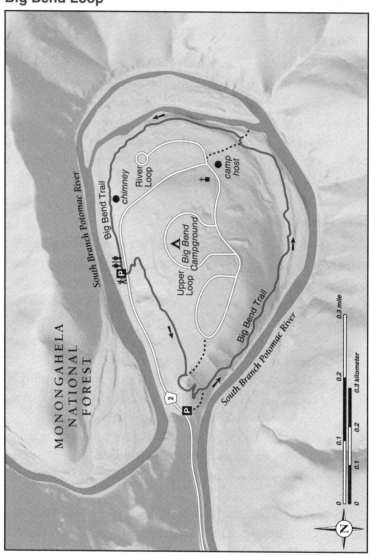

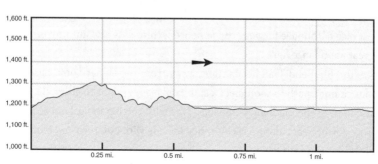

At 0.4 mile, a user-created trail leads right to an outcrop overlooking the river's edge. The South Branch Potomac River attracts not only hikers and campers but also anglers vying for trout and smallmouth bass. Around the campground and day-use area you will see folks fiddling with rods, hanging up waders, and telling fishing tales. However, even if you don't like to fish, this is a great destination. The setting can hardly be beat.

The Big Bend Trail drops to the water's edge and continues curving with the river. Enjoy views into the crystalline waterway, across which rise magnificent bluffs. After a little bit, the trail and river separate. Walk through thickets of pawpaw. They form an understory here and are often found together in groups because they reproduce by root sprouts. Pawpaws have large leaves, 6–12 inches in length, which droop like their tropical cousins farther south. Their yellow banana-like fruit are favored by wildlife, especially raccoons and opossums. Settlers made bread and pudding from pawpaw fruits. Farmers have attempted to cultivate pawpaws. Today a limited number of cultivars exist. Sycamores tower in the flat above the pawpaws. Wildflowers will be in abundance here in spring.

Enter a grassy clearing at 0.6 mile. You can see the campground maintenance area to your left. The open terrain also allows rewarding views of the surrounding walls of the Smoke Hole Canyon. Reenter flat woods of sycamore. At 0.8 mile, reach a trail junction. Here, a spur trail leads left to the River Loop of Big Bend Campground. The River Loop is set in a plain along the river. It was once a field and is growing up in white pine, sycamore, autumn olive, and a hodgepodge of other forest trees. Campsites are very dispersed. The U.S. Forest Service is keeping the area natural; many small trees and bushes provide dense cover and campsite privacy.

The Big Bend Trail splits right, then passes another spur leading out to the South Branch Potomac, which is splitting around an island. Continue downstream, circling behind the River Loop. Spur trails link the Big Bend Trail with individual campsites. A nearly sheer pine-clad bluff rises on the far side of the river. At 1.1 miles, pass the chimney of the old Ketterman Post Office, from the pre–Monongahela National Forest days. The final part of the circuit passes a restroom, then emerges at the parking area at 1.2 miles, completing the circuit.

Nearby Attractions

Big Bend Campground is set in the center of this hike and is a fine place to over-night in the Monongahela National Forest. It has 45 sites with water spigots and flush toilets. Campsites can be reserved online at recreation.gov.

Directions

From Petersburg, drive south on US 220 for 12.0 miles to County Road (CR) 2, which is just after a bridge crossing over South Branch Potomac River. Turn right on CR 2 and follow it 10.0 miles until it dead-ends at Big Bend Camp-ground. Park on the left, just before reaching the campground entrance gate.

THIS PART OF THE BIG BEND LOOP MAKES FOR EASY AND SCENIC HIKING.

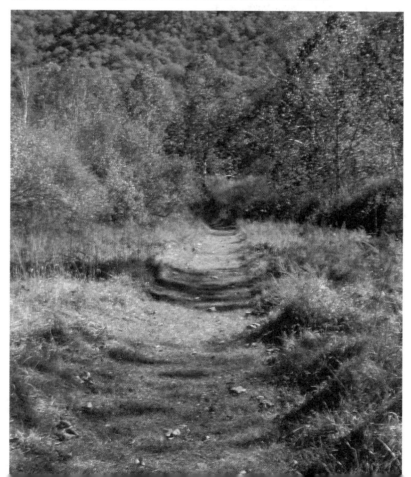

10 Seneca Rocks

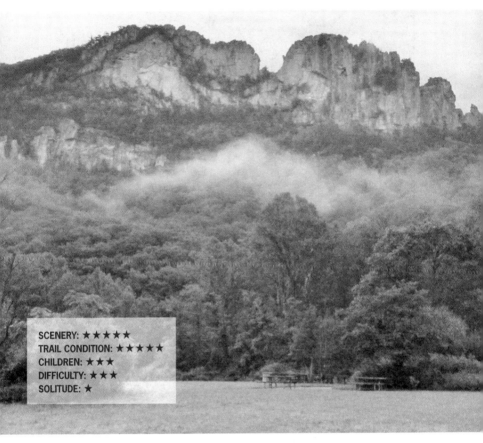

SCENERY: ★★★★★
TRAIL CONDITION: ★★★★★
CHILDREN: ★★★
DIFFICULTY: ★★★
SOLITUDE: ★

THE SENECA ROCKS FORM A JAGGED CREST AGAINST THE WEST VIRGINIA SKY.

GPS TRAILHEAD COORDINATES: N38° 50.040' W79° 22.454'

DISTANCE & CONFIGURATION: 3.2-mile out-and-back

HIKING TIME: 2 hours

HIGHLIGHTS: Seneca Rocks, Seneca Rocks Discovery Center, Sites Homestead, views

ELEVATION: 1,550' at trailhead, 2,360' at high point

ACCESS: No fees or permits required

MAPS: *Monongahela National Forest;* USGS *Upper Tract*

FACILITIES: Discovery center, homestead, picnic area, restrooms, water

WHEELCHAIR ACCESS: Yes, between discovery center and homestead

CONTACT: Cheat-Potomac Ranger District, 304-257-4488

Seneca Rocks

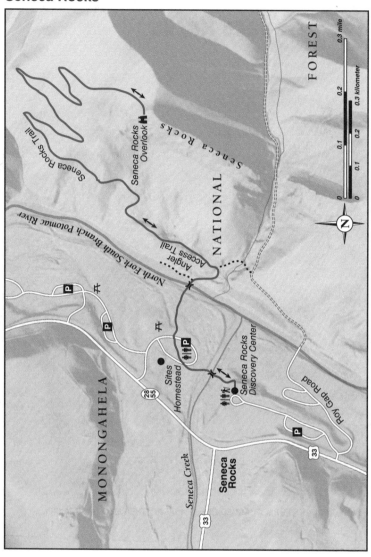

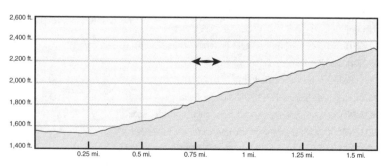

Overview

This hike starts at the fascinating Seneca Rocks Discovery Center, where you can learn all about the mountains of the Mountain State, then walk past the historic Sites Homestead before crossing the North Fork South Branch Potomac River on a big suspension bridge. From there, wind through incredible rock gardens. Finally, a series of switchbacks takes you to the Seneca Rocks, where an overlook and outcrops reveal views of the nearby valleys and ridges.

Route Details

Landmarks, by definition, stand out. However, some landmarks stand out more than others. The Seneca Rocks are one of West Virginia's most outstanding landmarks, and in the entire Appalachian range for that matter. These outcrops tower nearly 900 feet above the valley of the North Fork of the South Branch Potomac River. The pinnacles are very popular with rock climbers. We hikers can also visit those pinnacles without the risk associated with rock climbing via a well-maintained and graded foot trail to an observation platform, where the views are stunning. You can scramble beyond the viewing platform to more vistas atop the Seneca Rocks; however, it is officially discouraged—no wonder since 15 people have died falling from the Seneca Rocks since 1971. This includes climbers, but the message is the same—be careful up there.

The hike to Seneca Rocks is very popular, and the trail is designed to withstand many feet. However, you should respect the steep terrain over which the trail travels—please do not shortcut the switchbacks.

Despite what you may read on signs, it is not a 1,000-foot climb to the top, but merely a tad more than 800 feet. Nevertheless, many visitors will not make it to Seneca Rocks even though it is only 1.6 miles to the viewing platform and the trail is graded to ease the trek. Numerous trailside benches are available for resting. Hike this trail in the morning if possible—it is shady and cooler then.

Make sure to visit the Seneca Rocks Discovery Center before or after your hike. The human and natural history displays will enhance your understanding and appreciation of this slice of West Virginia. Start the trek behind the Seneca Rocks Discovery Center. A footpath leads left to a footbridge spanning rocky Seneca Creek. Open to a large parking area, the Sites Homestead comes into view and is worth a visit. Next, cross the parking area to the right, then come to a kiosk and trailhead. Here, join a wide path heading east through the woods. Seneca Rocks loom ahead, above the treeline.

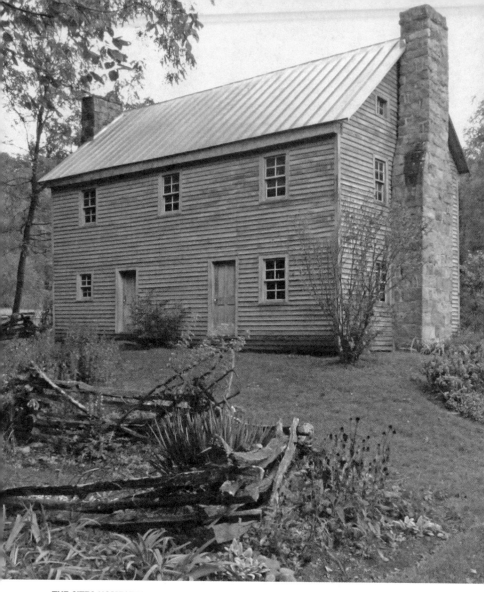

THE SITES HOMESTEAD, BUILT IN 1839, ADDS HISTORICAL INTEREST TO THE HIKE.

At 0.2 mile, reach a wide, long, and elaborate pedestrian bridge over the river. An angler access trail leaves left just after the bridge. The main gravel footpath continues right, curving past a rock outcrop. Trailside interpretive displays add more information about Seneca Rocks. At 0.3 mile, the trail splits. One path leads right to Roy Gap Road, crossing a perennial stream flowing off North Fork Mountain. Stay left with the Seneca Rocks Trail.

Notice the trail has been cleared of boulders that otherwise litter the oak-hickory forest. These boulders have fallen over time from the Seneca Rocks above. In places, fences must line the trail to discourage shortcuts despite more than adequate signage warning against shortcutting switchbacks. The climbing begins in earnest at 0.7 mile as the trail gains elevation via a series of steps. Next come many switchbacks, as the pathway rises as gradually as possible despite the very steep slope of the ridge below Seneca Rocks.

The Seneca Rocks are out of view as you angle up the mountainside. Keep climbing to a final series of steps, then reach an observation platform at 1.6 miles. From the platform, you can see west into the North Fork of the South Branch Potomac River, up the Seneca Creek valley, and the mountains that envelop them. North Fork Mountain stretches north. Look down to see where you came from and beyond. In the general platform area, you will see rock-climber trails and even a ranger-rescue road. In addition to the deadly falls from Seneca Rocks, rangers have to rescue injured hikers and climbers on an all-too-regular basis.

A rock promontory rises south from the platform. Climbing it is officially discouraged. However, extensive views stretch in all directions, especially up the North Fork valley. Be very careful if you go this route. The drop-offs are sheer and are recommended for rock climbers only. Do not walk one step beyond your capabilities. After looking out, you will appreciate the walk back down.

Nearby Attractions

This locale features not only the hike to Seneca Rocks but also the Seneca Rocks Discovery Center and the Sites Homestead. Built in 1839 and inhabited until 1947 by members of the Sites clan, the Sites Homestead was purchased by the U.S. Forest Service, then restored in 1989. It has since become an important part of interpreting the Seneca Rocks area. The house is open year-round to visit from the outside, and during the warm season occasional events are held at the house and on the grounds, where period gardens add historical flair.

Directions

From the intersection of US 33 and WV 28/55 in the town of Seneca Rocks, head south on US 33 0.5 mile, then turn left into the parking area for the Seneca Rocks Discovery Center. Seneca Rocks Trail starts in the rear of the discovery center.

Canaan Mountain Backcountry Circuit

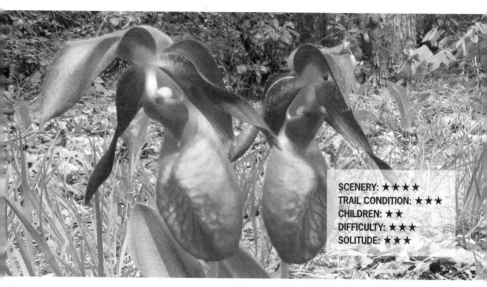

SCENERY: ★★★★
TRAIL CONDITION: ★★★
CHILDREN: ★★
DIFFICULTY: ★★★
SOLITUDE: ★★★

PINK LADY SLIPPERS ADORN THE RAILROAD GRADE TRAIL.

GPS TRAILHEAD COORDINATES: N39° 04.077' W79° 29.134'

DISTANCE & CONFIGURATION: 11.7-mile loop

HIKING TIME: 5.1 hours

HIGHLIGHTS: Trail shelters, waterfall

ELEVATION: 3,629' at trailhead, 4,112' at high point

ACCESS: No fees or permits required

MAPS: *Canaan Mountain Backcountry, Monongahela National Forest;* USGS *Blackwater Falls, Mozark Mountain*

FACILITIES: None

WHEELCHAIR ACCESS: None

CONTACT: Cheat-Potomac Ranger District, 304-257-4488

Overview

Explore this scenic, trail-rich mountaintop backcountry—perhaps even back-packing—complete with two trail shelters on the attractive route. First, circle toward Pointy Knob before turning into tumbling South Fork, reaching the first trail shelter, then running alongside dashing cascades and one cool waterfall.

From there, join the Railroad Grade Trail, passing yet another trail shelter. Finally, traverse deep forest back to the trailhead. Elevation changes aren't drastic, and this area receives much less use than nearby Dolly Sods.

Route Details

The Canaan Mountain Backcountry presents a fine trail network to execute loop hikes long and short. This particular hiking adventure can be enjoyed as a day hike or an overnight backpack, staying at one or both of the trail shelters encountered along the way. The well-marked and maintained trail network allows for trouble-free passage. And elevation changes of a 1,500-foot gain and a 1,500-foot loss spread over 11.7 miles of hiking make it very doable.

Leave the Allegheny Trail parking area and head west on Forest Road (FR) 13 for 0.3 mile, then turn left and join the Pointy Knob Trail (parking here is no good). A bumpy dead-end road enters the woods, and then you cut left on a blazed footpath rising from the dead end. Head south, rising amid spruce, red maple, and white pine. Quickly traverse a long double-planked boardwalk through spongy, mossy ground. Rise to rockier terrain, working toward the ridgecrest of Canaan Mountain. The narrow, brushy singletrack path winds amid windswept, almost stunted looking trees.

At 2.1 miles, the trail traverses an extremely rocky section. You are now running above 4,000 feet. At 2.6 miles, come along some rocks to your right and a high point. You can scramble around for partial views to the west of Canaan Valley State Park below.

From here, the Pointy Knob Trail drops off, then turns abruptly west, delving into the South Fork streamshed. Wander down though lightly wooded forest with scattered fern glades, contrasting with spruce thickets through which you otherwise pass. At 3.5 miles, step over the headwaters of South Fork, renewing the downgrade. Cross a wet meadow before reaching the South Run trail shelter at 3.9 miles. The three-sided wooden affair is set in a small clearing with a sizable wet meadow beyond. Water can be had from a stream downtrail beyond the shelter.

Descend the scenic South Fork valley, often well above the jaunty stream, dancing in perky cascades. Reach a pair of creek crossings at 5.1 miles. Cross again at 5.2 miles. You are now on the right bank, heading downstream in the deep, steep valley. At 5.4 miles, cross over to the left bank just above South Fork Falls, a 12-foot angled cataract that stairsteps to a long plunge pool. At 5.6 miles, rock-hop bigger Red Run, below where the South Fork and North Fork converge.

Canaan Mountain Backcountry

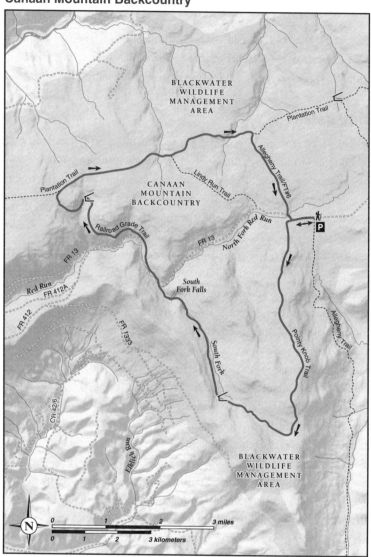

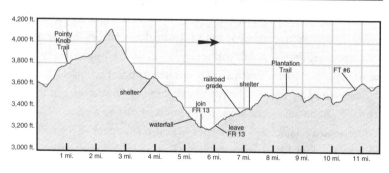

The trail turns upstream and rises to meet FR 13. Head left on the gravel road for 0.4 mile, paralleling Red Run, then split right with the signed Railroad Grade Trail at 6.1 miles. This path is relatively easy, but narrower than you may imagine, as it wanders under cherry, yellow birch, and beech trees. Circle a deeply incised tributary valley of Red Creek, reaching a trail shelter and stream at 7.4 miles. Here, the Adirondack-style refuge is wonderfully perched just above a small spring branch and shaded by hardwoods and evergreens. A picnic table and fire ring complement the scene.

The Railroad Grade Trail crosses the bouldery stream to soon meet the Plantation Trail at 7.9 miles. Here, head right in spruce-dominated woods. The Plantation Trail got its name after the Civilian Conservation Corps (CCC) planted red spruce here. The original forest was logged from 1890 to 1910. Terrible fires followed the logging before the area became part of the Monongahela National Forest. Now we travel east among completely recovered and majestic woodland belying the logging of yesteryear. Work around occasional boggy spots, then descend to cross a pair of branches forming Lindy Run.

At 9.3 miles, intersect the Lindy Run Trail as it shortcuts right to FR 13. Stay easterly with the Plantation Trail, bisecting a rocky section amid heath with low-slung mountain laurel and rhododendron. Dip to cross Shays Run, then rise to meet Fire Trail #6, with which the Allegheny Trail runs in conjunction. When the CCC cut in the fire roads, they numbered the roads in sequence. Most of these old roads have returned to seed. From here, gently rise south over another rocky segment with low-slung vegetation, then drop to reach FR 13 at 11.4 miles. Turn left on the gravel road to reach the trailhead, completing the hike at 11.7 miles.

Nearby Attractions

Miles of pathways linking the Canaan Mountain trails of the Monongahela National Forest to other federal, state, and local paths around Davis and Thomas have been constructed. For more information on Tucker County's huge local trail network, visit the Heart of the Highlands Trail System at heartofthehighlandstrail.org.

Directions

From the town of Davis, drive south on WV 32 for 3.3 miles to Canaan Loop Road. Turn right on Canaan Loop Road (which becomes FR 13) and follow it 3.9 miles to the Allegheny Trail parking area, on your left. Begin the hike by walking west on FR 13 for 0.3 mile, then veering left onto Pointy Knob Trail.

12 Table Rock Overlook

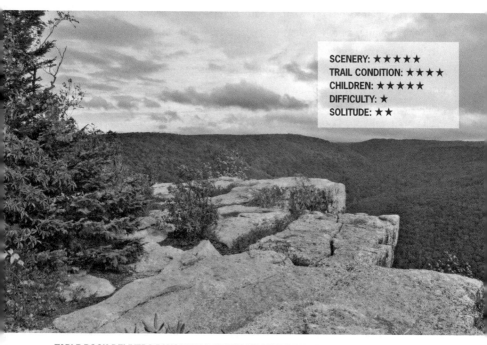

SCENERY: ★★★★
TRAIL CONDITION: ★★★★
CHILDREN: ★★★★★
DIFFICULTY: ★
SOLITUDE: ★★

TABLE ROCK DELIVERS PANORAMAS OF THE DRY FORK VALLEY BELOW.

GPS TRAILHEAD COORDINATES: N39° 03.916' W79° 34.399'

DISTANCE & CONFIGURATION: 2.2-mile out-and-back

HIKING TIME: 1–1.5 hours

HIGHLIGHTS: Expansive vista, rock climbing

ELEVATION: 3,315' at trailhead, 3,405' at high point

ACCESS: No fees or permits required

MAPS: *Monongahela National Forest;* USGS *Mozark Mountain*

FACILITIES: None

WHEELCHAIR ACCESS: None

CONTACT: Cheat-Potomac Ranger District, 304-478-3251

Overview

This easy hike reaps great rewards. Table Rock Trail (Forest Trail #113) leads to the craggy southwestern edge of Canaan Mountain, a high-elevation plateau featuring flora and fauna more like Canada than West Virginia. Be forewarned that the Table Rock outcrop has some big crevasses in it, so keep the kids close while taking in the great view of the Red Run and Dry Fork of Cheat River valleys. Those same crevasses and sheer cliffs of Table Rock attract technical rock climbers who may be plying their trade from the overlook.

Route Details

This trail was the first hike I ever did in the Monongahela National Forest. I remember it well—the rich forest, the high-country aromas, and especially the view from the flat expanse of Table Rock. The experience has drawn me back again, and I still consider it one of the Monongahela's finest overlooks.

Table Rock Trail is part of the Canaan (pronounced: ka-nane) Mountain Backcountry, in the Potomac Highlands near the Dolly Sods as well as Blackwater River State Park. Thus, Canaan Mountain Backcountry receives light hiking pressure, due to these other destinations sucking away visitors. But do not overlook this fine parcel of the Monongahela National Forest, especially Table Rock Overlook. Canaan Mountain is a plateau with elevations ranging from 3,100 feet to 4,145 feet. The trails are gentle throughout the plateau, dotted with three Adirondack-style trail shelters among its pathway network.

Canaan Mountain was first logged from 1890 to 1910. Terrible wildfires followed the logging. The mountaintop was then purchased by the U.S. Department of Agriculture, subsequently becoming part of the Monongahela National Forest. In an effort to rehabilitate Canaan Mountain, the 1930s Great Depression–era work relief program, the Civilian Conservation Corps (CCC), planted red spruce to replace the logged woodlands. When it did, the CCC also planned hiking trails and fire roads. These same CCC tracks are used today as part of the Canaan Mountain Backcountry.

Start this hike from Canaan Loop Road, a scenic drive in and of itself, passing several trailheads. However, the northern part of the loop road crosses into private land and is under-maintained and therefore not recommended unless you are interested in getting your vehicle stuck on a mountaintop and seeing what happens next. The Table Rock Trail enters a forest of beech, black cherry, maple, and yellow birch. Scattered rhododendron thickets add a touch of year-round evergreen. The marked trail is nearly level, then angles up the side of a hill, rising to your left. It soon levels again—overall elevation variances are only a little more than 100 feet between high and low points, so the hike ends up being level far more than not. Below you are mosses, ferns, and a lot of rocks.

Table Rock Overlook

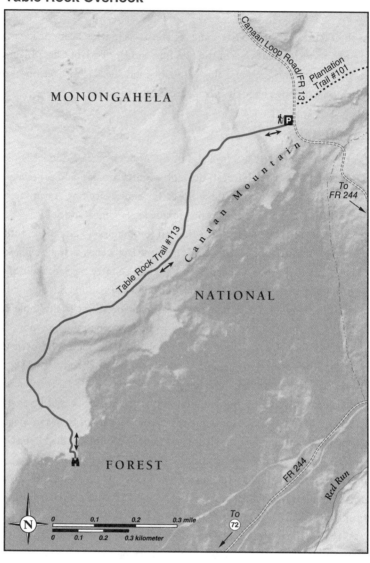

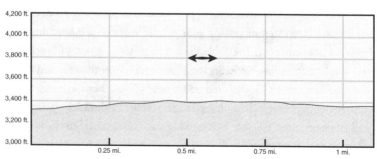

At 0.5 mile, the trail descends a bit, then enters a rhododendron thicket that is muddy in spots. The trail then turns a little more southwest as you pick your way along the muck. Try to stay on the path—if you walk on the edge of the wet area, the wet area will only widen. In many spots, trail engineers have constructed rock and wood trail beds to secure dry passage through the mire.

Come to a campsite just before opening onto Table Rock at 1.1 miles. Here, the trail splits. The primary trail goes left to an outcrop. Here, a large, level rock face opens to the Dry Fork gorge below. Dwarf spruce, mountain laurel, and brush fight to make a living in small fissures of Table Rock. More substantial crevasses open at your feet and must be accounted for. Green Mountain stands across from you, to the southeast, separated by the gulf of Red Run. A spruce forest resides atop Green Mountain and is surrounded by hardwoods.

Still another path opens to the largest part of the sandstone surface that is Table Rock, so named for the flatness of its top. To the southwest, Green Mountain and the Otter Creek Wilderness stand in untamed grandeur. Below, the Dry Fork of the Cheat River flows west through a rampart of highlands. Downstream, see where Otter Creek cuts its vale, meeting Dry Fork.

As you work your way around the outcrops, carefully notice how much these ledges overhang the depths below. Look down from Table Rock and observe how some boulders could not stand the test of time, falling to the forest below. Some of the crevasses are 100 feet or more deep. Watch your footing, then find a good spot to take it all in. While out here you might see some roped-in climbers challenging the sheer drop-offs.

Nearby Attractions

The Canaan Backcountry, accessible from the road to this hike, presents more than 13,000 acres of wild mountain splendor laced with hiking trails for further exploration. The trails here link with adjacent Blackwater Falls State Park and Canaan Valley State Park, two additional worthy West Virginia destinations. As its name suggests, Blackwater Falls is known for its cascades and cataracts, while Canaan Valley is more a resort-type state park.

Directions

From the town of Davis, drive south on WV 32 for 3.3 miles to Canaan Loop Road. Turn right on Canaan Loop Road and follow it 9.8 miles to the Table Rock Trail on your left.

Blackwater Canyon Trail

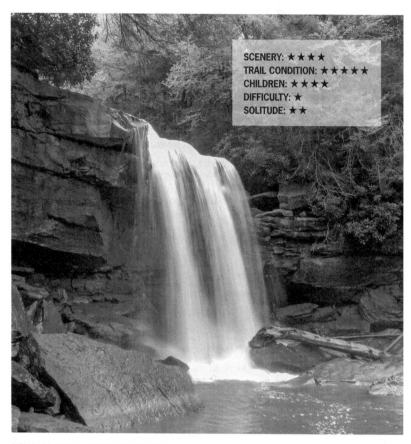

SCENERY: ★★★★
TRAIL CONDITION: ★★★★★
CHILDREN: ★★★★
DIFFICULTY: ★
SOLITUDE: ★★

DOUGLAS FALLS MAKES ITS PLUNGE.

GPS TRAILHEAD COORDINATES: N39° 07.515' W79° 31.126'

DISTANCE & CONFIGURATION: 1.8-mile out-and-back

HIKING TIME: 1.0 hours

HIGHLIGHTS: Douglas Falls, Kennedy Falls

ELEVATION: 2,774' at trailhead, 2,652' at low point

ACCESS: No fees or permits required

MAPS: *Monongahela National Forest;* USGS *Lead Mine, Mozark Mountain*

FACILITIES: None

WHEELCHAIR ACCESS: None

CONTACT: Cheat-Potomac Ranger District, 304-257-4488

Overview

Explore the history of the mining town of Douglas before embarking on a converted rail-trail, visiting easy-to-reach Douglas Falls and, if you choose, more difficult to access Kennedy Falls. Trace the wide, easy, and nearly level rail-trail to the confluence of North Fork Blackwater River and the Blackwater River. After your hike, check out the nearby funky mountain towns of Thomas and Davis.

Route Details

The canyons of the North Fork Blackwater River and the Blackwater River, where this trek takes place, are spectacular natural assets. Portions of the canyons were purchased by the Monongahela National Forest, while other parts were bought by the state of West Virginia, turning their section into worth-a-visit Blackwater Falls State Park. In 1983, the rail line through the Blackwater River canyon—once carrying timber, coal, and coke—was deactivated. The U.S. Forest Service turned the track into a rail-trail, even though the old rail line itself forms the forest boundary with a private timber interest.

Today, the Blackwater Canyon Trail runs 10.5 miles from Thomas to Hendricks, dropping over 1,000 feet along the way. (It's about 8 miles to Hendricks from the trailhead for this hike.) Our hike explores a portion of the trek. When the line was operating, multiple engines were necessary to move product up or down the steep canyon. Before the 1880s, this area was the back of beyond, before Henry Davis—for whom the adjacent town of Davis is named—bought vast virgin tracts of land and then hauled the wood out by the marvel of a railroad. Coal interests followed, with coke ovens built, converting the coal into coke (a very pure form of carbon used to smelt iron into steel). The boomtown of Douglas sprang up around the trailhead for this hike. Along the last part of the drive to the trailhead, stop and soak in the interpretive information about life in this coal/coke/lumber town. See the brick "beehive" ovens used to make coke.

In the early 1900s, Douglas, Davis, and Thomas held over 5,000 residents. Then the forests came down, and the coal mines were deepened. Even the coke ovens were cooled as a more efficient process of making coke came to be. The area went into decline, despite some coal mining still being undertaken. The communities hit a low point before interest in this combination of mountains, the huge perched Canaan Valley, and canyons came to be recognized as a superior natural asset. The now-preserved area is laced with trails. The towns cater to visitors coming to enjoy this natural mountain splendor.

Blackwater Canyon Trail

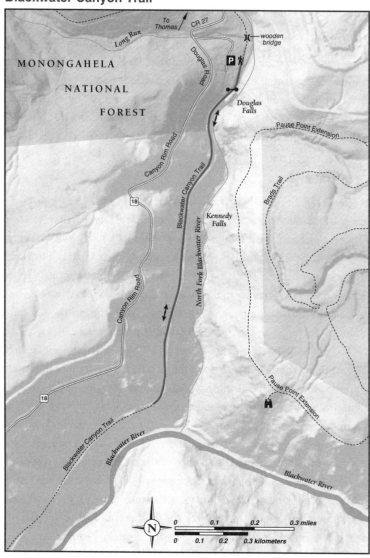

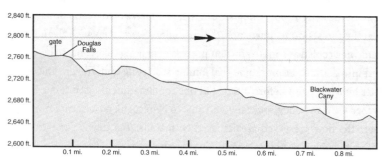

And you will see some of that splendor on this trek, as well as some of the negative aftereffects of mining. Leave the parking area on a wide track, passing a house on your right. North Fork Blackwater River flows to your left. Note the orange-tinted rocks, evidence of acid mine runoff that has made some stretches too acidic for aquatic life. However, the area mines have been reclaimed. Pass a low slide cascade. At 0.1 mile, reach a U.S. Forest Service gate. Drop left along a rock rampart just beyond the gate to reach the base of Douglas Falls, where you will see the banks have been stabilized. Here, Douglas Falls makes a 30-foot dive, widening as it descends into an aqua plunge pool.

From there, return to the rail-trail and continue downriver. At 0.4 mile, look left for a faint but usually marked user-created trail dropping to Kennedy Falls. It's a rough go down to the 30-or-so-foot spiller, making its own stair-step plunge off a rim into another pool. Daredevil kayakers paddling the North Fork claim an earlier name for this cataract—Gluteas Mash. By any name, the waterfall is worth the side trip.

Returning to the Blackwater Canyon Trail, continue cruising south until at 0.9 mile you come to where the canyons of the North Fork and Blackwater River converge. Even through the trees you can recognize the mountain cleft widening. This is a good place to turn around, with only 120 feet to climb back to the trailhead. Hopefully you burned enough calories to justify a dining and touring experience in nearby Davis or Thomas.

Nearby Attractions

Davis and Thomas are two former logging and mining towns reinvented as hiker, skier, and bicycler mountain towns aimed at entertaining visitors.

Directions

From downtown Thomas, take WV 32 north 0.1 mile, then turn right onto Douglas Road/County Road (CR) 27 and follow it for 1.0 mile. Veer left onto Rail Falls Road (CR 27/3) and follow it 1.0 mile to end at a parking area on the left, just after the primitive wooden bridge over Long Run. The bridge is a little rough, and be apprised there is a parking area just before the bridge.

Lower Otter
Creek Wilderness

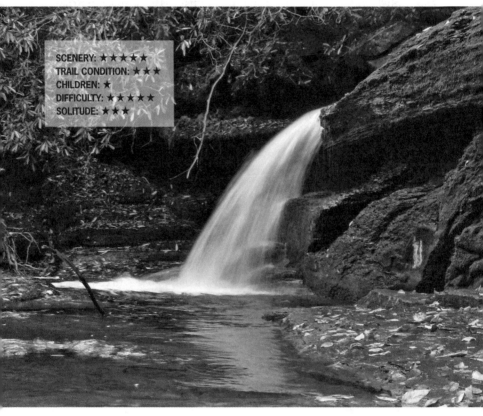

SCENERY: ★★★★★
TRAIL CONDITION: ★★★
CHILDREN: ★
DIFFICULTY: ★★★★★
SOLITUDE: ★★★

OTTER CREEK FALLS LIES DEEP IN WILDERNESS.

GPS TRAILHEAD COORDINATES: N39° 02.671' W79° 36.418'

DISTANCE & CONFIGURATION: 14.2-mile out-and-back

HIKING TIME: 7.5 hours

HIGHLIGHTS: Remoteness, waterfalls, wilderness

ELEVATION: 1,840' at trailhead, 2,750' at high point

ACCESS: No fees or permits required

MAPS: *Otter Creek Wilderness, Monongahela National Forest;* USGS *Mozark Mountain, Parsons, Bowden*

FACILITIES: None

WHEELCHAIR ACCESS: None

CONTACT: Cheat-Potomac Ranger District, 304-478-3251

Overview

This hike starts in the lowermost part of Otter Creek Wilderness, then delves deep into the Otter Creek valley, viewing first-rate aquatic scenery, including a few waterfalls that enhance an everywhere-you-look beauty deserving of its wilderness status. First, cross Dry Fork on a huge suspension bridge, then join an old railroad grade, slowly gaining elevation. The hike crosses scenic tributaries and visits three attractive yet differing sets of falls, culminating in Otter Creek Falls. Though elevation changes are slight, it is still a 14-mile out-and-back hike.

Route Details

Otter Creek is the star of the show on this hike. Though this gorgeous mountain valley was logged and homesteaded a century back, it has been under federal protection since 1917 when the watershed was acquired as a preserved water supply, and later became a part of the Monongahela National Forest. The state of West Virginia established a limestone neutralization plant at the headwaters of Otter Creek in 1964 to make the stream less acidic and improve the conditions for native brook trout. Though parts of the valley were later logged, most of the area was spared and the Otter Creek Wilderness was established in 1975. Today, the area is a wilderness in the truest sense of the word. Take your time, noticing the vegetation variety while looking for wildlife from black bears to grouse. Also, look for the many pools and cascades of Otter Creek in addition to those noted on this hike.

Leave the parking area on the Otter Creek Trail and enter the woods on a gated forest road. Wind down to Dry Fork, then cross this river on an elaborate suspension footbridge. Immediately turn right and follow Dry Fork downstream just a bit, reaching an Otter Creek Wilderness sign at 0.2 mile. Turn left, go up the steps, join a footpath and parallel Otter Creek upstream, working through irregular terrain. Do not cross Otter Creek here.

Pass a small waterfall dripping from a bluff to your left, then walk by the foundations of an old homesite. Hop Coal Run at 0.9 mile. Trace a railroad grade upstream beneath a tall forest of tulip trees. These trees are present at lower elevations in the Central Appalachians. The elevation here is just more than 1,800 feet, very low by Monongahela National Forest standards.

The railroad grade stays nearly level and straight, making for easy hiking. Old clearings and fields are all but gone these days, replaced by ferns, trees, and some patches of rhododendron. Otter Creek sings to your right as it slaloms

Lower Otter Creek Wilderness

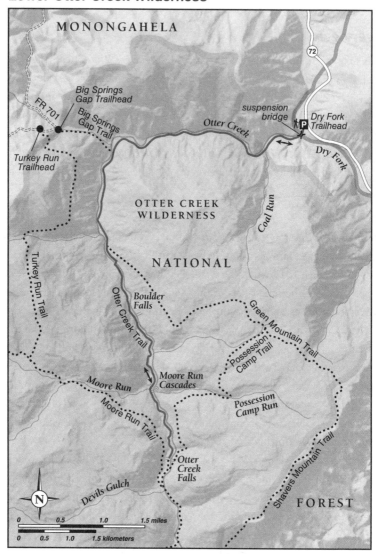

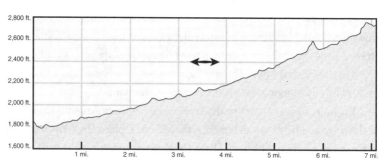

through giant boulders. Ironically, in autumn lower stream segments will run underground, appearing dried up. At 2.0 miles, traverse an area where the railroad grade was cut through a hill. A sheer bluff rises across the stream. Spur trails lead to campsites. At 2.5 miles, a bluff on your left and the creek to your right pinch in the trail. Make a sweeping turn south at 2.8 miles, then reach a trail junction at 3.0 miles. Piles of rocks, called cairns, mark this junction and all others in this wilderness. Here, Big Springs Gap Trail leaves west on a long crossing of tan-colored Otter Creek, then rises away to McGowan Mountain.

Stay straight on the Otter Creek Trail, which becomes pinched in once again by low, attractive bluffs. This section of stream features a series of alluring swimming and fishing holes, and is pocked with big boulders good for sunning. At 4.2 miles, the Green Mountain Trail splits off to your left at a V intersection. Keep straight on the Otter Creek Trail, skirting through rhododendron patches.

At 4.5 miles, reach a campsite and crossing of Otter Creek. This likely wet ford crosses over to a sand beach. Keep heading upstream, rising far above the river now flowing to your left. The rhododendron thickens, and the trail squeezes by a bluff at 4.8 miles. Railroad ties are visible in the trailbed. Work your way through some sloped landslide areas. Look for Boulder Falls, well below the trail, at 5.2 miles. Here, Otter Creek spills about 10 feet over a boulder-bordered ledge into a long pool lined with yet more boulders. To reach the falls you have to go downstream a bit to avoid a bluff, then fight your way through rhododendron. Most hikers only gaze down on the cataract from the trail.

Continue upstream, stepping away briefly from the grade at 5.7 miles. Reach Moore Run at mile 6.1. It is a rock-hop crossing. Here, a wide rock outcrop stretches to the confluence of Moore Run and Otter Creek. At the confluence, Otter Creek slides about 10 feet over a layered rock face, creating Moore Run Cascades. Adjacent rock slabs make for sunny observation platforms unless the water is high and flowing over the slabs.

The Otter Creek Trail passes beside a campsite and continues upstream. It next leaves the grade at 6.8 miles, climbs through rocky woods, then returns to the railroad grade at 7.0 miles. Pass a rock bluff to the right of the trail. At 7.1 miles, the trail comes to Otter Creek Falls. Here, the dark stream tumbles 12 feet over a rhododendron-bordered ledge. Depending on weather, the spill can be a single channel at lower water levels or wider when Otter Creek is up. The stream splashes onto a wide rock slab and continues downstream. This slab affords photography spots, as does the trailside terrain above the falls. If you reach the intersection with Moore Run Trail and Possession Camp Trail, you have gone too far. Remember, it is a full 7.1 miles back to the trailhead.

Nearby Attractions

Otter Creek Wilderness presents 45 miles of hiking trails within its 20,000-acre boundaries. Accessible from seven trailheads, elevations range from 1,800 feet at the start of this hike to more than 3,900 feet. Therefore, the locale has lots of pathways and terrain to explore, especially if you are willing to backpack.

Directions

From downtown Parsons, head north on US 219 for 2.0 miles to WV 72. Turn right on WV 72 and follow it 4.4 miles to the Dry Fork Trailhead. This will be a signed right turn onto a gravel road, leading to the actual parking area.

THIS BRIDGE LEADS YOU INTO THE OTTER CREEK WILDERNESS.

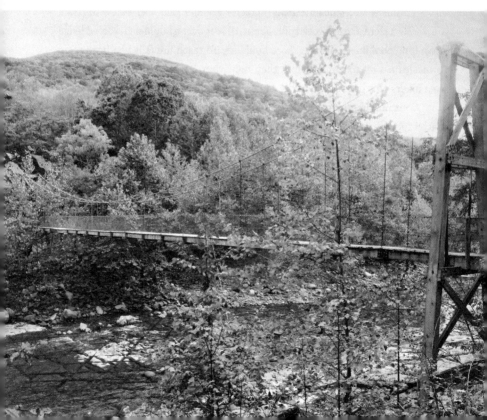

Otter Creek
Wilderness Loop

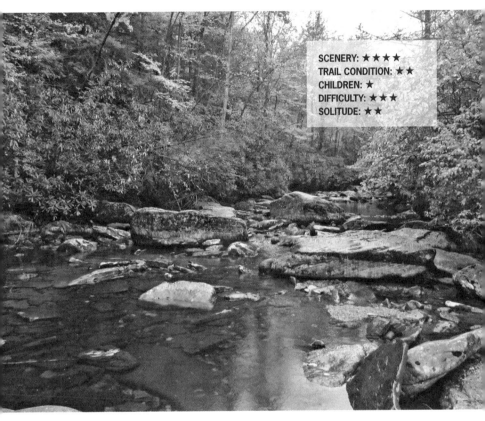

SCENERY: ★ ★ ★ ★
TRAIL CONDITION: ★ ★
CHILDREN: ★
DIFFICULTY: ★ ★ ★
SOLITUDE: ★ ★

THE BOULDER-STREWN CROSSING OF OTTER CREEK ON THE MYLIUS TRAIL

GPS TRAILHEAD COORDINATES: N38° 56.475' W79° 40.117'

DISTANCE & CONFIGURATION: 8.7-mile loop

HIKING TIME: 5 hours

HIGHLIGHTS: Some views, streams, wilderness

ELEVATION: 3,010' at trailhead, 3,840' at high point

ACCESS: No fees or permits required

MAPS: *Otter Creek Wilderness, Monongahela National Forest;* USGS *Bowden*

FACILITIES: None

WHEELCHAIR ACCESS: None

CONTACT: Cheat-Potomac Ranger District, 304-478-3251

Otter Creek Wilderness Loop

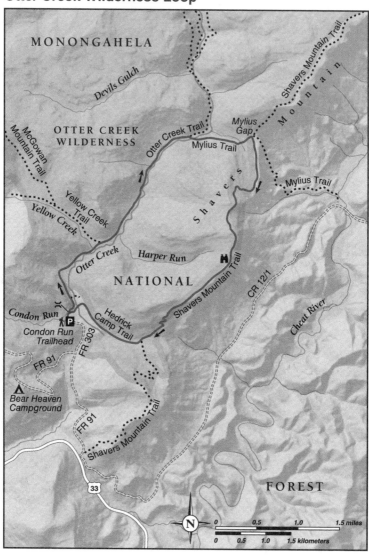

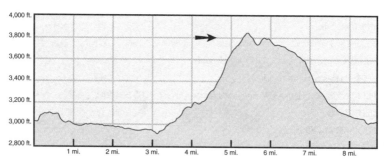

Overview

This loop explores the high and the low of the Otter Creek Wilderness. Trace Otter Creek from its headwaters as it cascades down the valley, gathering in pools, down to where it gets big enough for swimming holes. Then climb out of the valley to Mylius Gap atop Shavers Mountain. Make a solid climb to a high point on Shavers Mountain. Enjoy some views and ridgetop walking before returning to the Otter Creek valley via the Hedrick Camp Trail. There will be other hikers along Otter Creek, but after that you should relish in solitude.

Route Details

This is a true wilderness hike. The trails are primitive, albeit well used, and trail junctions are marked with simple rock cairns rather than signs. Therefore, map-reading and navigational skills will help. So will a GPS. Furthermore, once atop Shavers Mountain, old roads and private roads split from the main trail, creating potential confusion. Just stay with the hiking trails, don't drop east into the Glady Fork valley, and you will be fine. Campsites are abundant on Otter Creek but are limited after Mylius Gap.

Leave the Condon Run Trailhead and follow the gated road to a footbridge. Your return route, Hedrick Camp Trail, comes in through a rhododendron thicket to your right just before the footbridge. Cross Condon Run, skirt a field, and continue on the forest road. This road leads down to a limestone treatment plant constructed to reduce acidity in Otter Creek and improve fish habitat. Stay on the road for 0.2 mile, then split left on the Otter Creek Trail, entering the wilderness proper as the forest road descends right. Follow an old logging grade flanked by rhododendron.

Come alongside Otter Creek at 0.8 mile, as it flows through a mix of meadows and woods. Enter a meadow at 1.0 mile. An old railroad bridge abutment is alongside Otter Creek. Soak in upstream vistas here. Turn left, tracing the grade and stepping over sandy Yellow Creek at 1.1 miles. Enter evergreen woods, then find the Yellow Creek Trail at 1.2 miles. A cairn of stones marks this junction, like others in this wilderness.

Keep forward on the Otter Creek Trail. Note the embedded railroad ties in the path as rhododendron closes in on the route. Many dry streambeds come in from your left, resulting in dips in the rail grade. At 2.1 miles, climb a bit, skirting a cabin-size boulder.

Drop to the grade briefly, then veer right at another clearing. Red Creek is just a few feet away at 2.2 miles. Mountain laurel and rhododendron crowd the path as the canopy opens overhead. Step over a feeder branch of Otter Creek at 2.4 miles. Otter Creek is nearby, flowing loudly among rocks and boulders. Rejoin the grade as it becomes very mucky. Take the trail up and to your left, bypassing the mess.

Pass near a clearing, drop back down to the rail grade, and then intersect the Mylius Trail at 3.1 miles. This is a lesser-evident trail junction, so keep on your toes. Turn right (east) on the Mylius Trail, dropping a bit into a rhododendron thicket. Pass a campsite, then reach a boulder-strewn crossing of Otter Creek. Ford the stream, continuing on the Mylius Trail and making a mild and shady upgrade. Step over a stream at 3.7 miles, your last water for a long time. Reach Mylius Gap and a campsite on Shavers Mountain at 3.9 miles. Turn right here, following the Shavers Mountain Trail south.

The forest here is mixed, with drier species such as oak interspersed with Fraser magnolia and northern hardwoods. The climb is easy at first, and levels out, passing a property boundary marker at 4.6 miles. Next, begin switchbacking steeply up Shavers Mountain, often going where you think the trail won't or shouldn't go, staying inside the national forest boundary. Top out at 5.4 miles, after climbing 700 feet from Mylius Gap.

You are back on the ridgecrest. You will immediately lose elevation as you reach a gap at 5.7 miles. Climb a second knob. You are on the edge of the Shavers Mountain escarpment. At 5.8 miles, head to the eastern mountainside, grabbing views of the Glady Fork valley and Middle Mountain. Be careful here, as doubletrack primitive roads coming in from the east can tempt you off the singletrack Shavers Mountain Trail.

You are now heading southwest as the trail makes an easy downgrade. At 6.9 miles, in a brushy area, make the first of four switchbacks downhill. The path alternates between rocks and wet places. Intersect the Hedrick Camp Trail at 7.4 miles. Shavers Mountain Trail veers up and away to your left. Stay straight on the rhododendron-bordered Hedrick Camp Trail as it travels an old grade. Come alongside the headwaters of Otter Creek in a widening flat. Leave the grade at 8.4 miles, dropping left into rhododendron. Soon cross Otter Creek on a primitive log bridge in an area flooded by beavers. Gently ascend from Otter Creek. Condon Run flows on your right. Emerge onto the closed forest road near the Condon Run Trailhead. Turn left on the closed forest road, walk a few feet, and reach the Condon Run Trailhead, completing your loop at mile 8.7.

Nearby Attractions

Stuart Memorial Drive/Forest Road (FR) 91 travels along the south side of the Otter Creek Wilderness. It extends 10.0 miles, linking the Elkins area with Otter Creek. Along the way, it passes numerous recreation sites, including Bear Heaven Campground.

Directions

From Elkins, drive east on US 33 for 11.5 miles to Stuart Memorial Drive/ FR 91 at Alpena Gap on Shavers Mountain. Turn left on FR 91 (if you reach County Road 12 you've gone too far) and follow it 1.1 miles to a junction. Stay forward at the junction, now on FR 303, and dead-end at the Condon Run Trailhead in 0.4 mile.

Seneca Creek Backcountry–Laurel Fork Wilderness Area

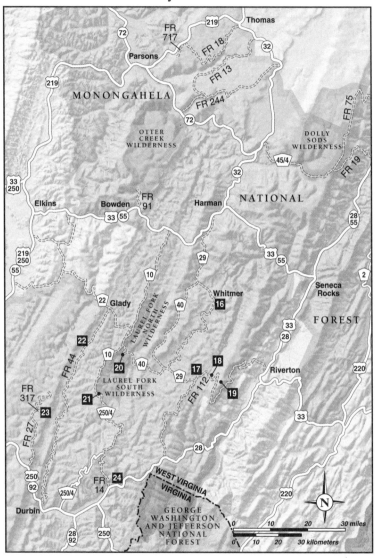

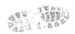

Seneca Creek Backcountry– Laurel Fork Wilderness Area

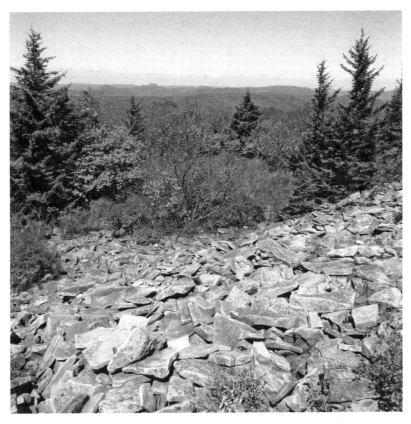

SOAK IN THIS VIEW OF SENECA CREEK BACKCOUNTRY. *(See Hike 19, page 101.)*

Horton–Spring Ridge Loop

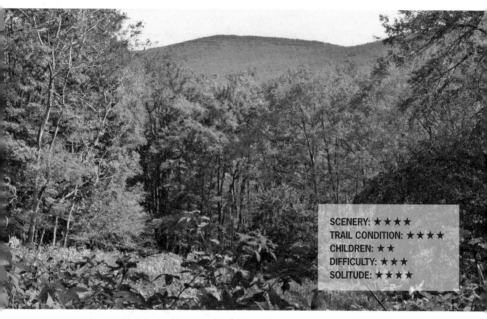

A SLOPED MEADOW OPENS TO A VISTA OF SPRUCE MOUNTAIN.

> SCENERY: ★ ★ ★ ★
> TRAIL CONDITION: ★ ★ ★ ★
> CHILDREN: ★ ★
> DIFFICULTY: ★ ★ ★
> SOLITUDE: ★ ★ ★ ★

GPS TRAILHEAD COORDINATES: N38° 47.911' W79° 32.675'

DISTANCE & CONFIGURATION: 6.8-mile loop

HIKING TIME: 3.5 hours

HIGHLIGHTS: Diverse environments, views, wildlife

ELEVATION: 2,850' at trailhead, 4,140' at high point

ACCESS: No fees or permits required

MAPS: *Seneca Creek Backcountry, Monongahela National Forest; USGS Whitmer*

FACILITIES: None

WHEELCHAIR ACCESS: None

CONTACT: Cheat-Potomac Ranger District, 304-257-4488

Overview

This classic stream and ridge loop hike ascends very pretty Lower Two Spring Run valley along an old wagon road that formerly linked the hamlets of Horton on Gandy Creek and Riverton on South Branch Potomac River. Join the Allegheny Mountain Trail to bisect a mountainside meadow where evergreen-topped mountains are the centerpieces of a fine view. Next, take the Spring Ridge Trail through wildlife clearings aplenty. Your return trip to Gandy Creek is a pleasant woodland stroll. Though the grades are not terribly steep, there are few level sections along this hike that ends with a short road walk to complete the circuit.

Route Details

This is the lowest elevation trailhead of the entire Seneca Creek Backcountry, leaving you a nearly 1,300-foot climb to the hike's high point. Depart the parking area and quickly join the Horton Trail, named for the nearby community of Horton. Come alongside Lower Two Spring Run, a smallish stream in a deep valley draining west down Allegheny Mountain. Follow the old road along the right bank of the stream. At 0.2 mile, briefly leave the road, circumventing a washed-out area.

Continue up the rocky valley, which lies beneath a hardwood forest with a light understory. Note how the south-facing side of the valley is rife with oak while the north-facing side of the valley has more moss, evergreen, and birch. It is simply a matter of exposure.

This trail is a good place to discern between yellow birch and black birch trees. Yellow birch, found frequently throughout the Monongahela, are easy to spot. They have a yellowish-gold bark with horizontal stripes. The ragged bark peels on the tree. However, larger yellow birch will not have bark peeling on their lower trunks, but will still have peeling bark on their upper branches. Black birch, also known as sweet birch, is less common and has horizontal stripes on the bark, which is more brownish-gray. The bark does not peel; it is tight and resembles that of a cherry tree. Scratch a twig of black birch and it smells like wintergreen. In the Monongahela, black birch grow in moist areas along lower-elevation mountain streams.

Bypass another washout at 0.4 mile. Some oaks in the lower valley are big. Cross Lower Two Spring Run at 0.6 mile and 0.9 mile, once again picking up the roadbed. Stay directly alongside the stream, which drops steeply, resulting in numerous eye-pleasing yet modest cascades. Cross the stream twice more at mile 1.1. You are now on the right bank. At 1.6 miles, the Horton Trail now reaches a fork in Lower Two Spring Run. Curve right (southeast) alongside the right fork. The trail rises sharply as you step back and forth over the small stream, then meet the Allegheny Mountain Trail at 2.5 miles.

Turn right on the Allegheny Mountain Trail and walk just a few feet to another trail junction. Here, the Horton Trail leaves left down to Seneca Creek,

Horton–Spring Ridge Loop

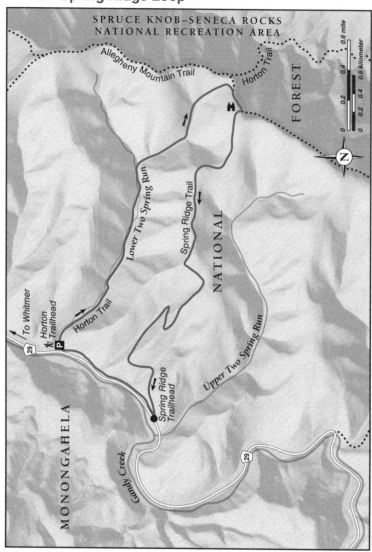

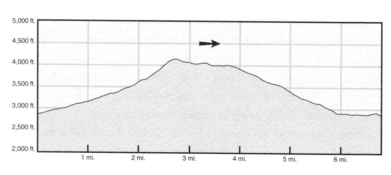

finding the Upper Falls of Seneca. Stay right, climbing on the Allegheny Mountain Trail. Enter a sloped wildlife clearing. Make sure and look back for a view of the north end of Spruce Mountain. Reenter woods just before coming to a third trail junction at 2.7 miles. Turn acutely right, joining the Spring Ridge Trail.

This wide, grassy lane makes for easy walking. Drop moderately to a small clearing at 3.2 miles. These meadows and edges of woods and fields make for good wildlife viewing opportunities. I've seen deer and bears on this loop. The trail then levels off and passes another clearing at 3.4 miles. Watch for the remains of a wildlife-watering pond at 3.8 miles. At 4.0 miles, slip over to the right-hand side of the ridge and keep descending. Partial views of the Gandy Creek valley and Middle Mountain open to your right.

At 4.6 miles, switchback to the right, then to the left, entering a rocky cove. Parallel a small stream on the right side of the trail. The path drops sharply then levels off as the stream continues to descend. At 5.3 miles, pass a castlelike rock outcrop to your left. Slip in and out of a small hollow. Gandy Creek becomes audible below. Reach County Road (CR) 29 at 5.9 miles. Turn right on the gravel road and mostly descend, coming to the Horton Trail parking area at 6.8 miles, completing your loop.

Nearby Attractions

On the way to the trailhead you pass Spruce Knob Lake Campground, the highest campground in West Virginia, next to the highest lake in the state, and the highest point in the state. Make this your base camp to explore the trails of the Seneca Creek Backcountry, including the Horton–Spring Ridge Loop. Campers can enjoy the cool air of the high country at drive-up campsites or walk-in tent campsites.

Directions

From the town of Seneca Rocks, head south on US 33 for 13.0 miles to Briery Gap Road. Turn right on Briery Gap Road and follow it up 2.5 miles to Forest Road (FR) 112. Turn right on FR 112 and head up 13.2 miles to FR 1. Turn right on FR 1 and follow it 4.1 miles to CR 29. Stay right and follow CR 29 for 9.3 miles to a parking area on your right.

Alternate directions: From the hamlet of Whitmer, take CR 29 south 1.3 miles to the trailhead on your left.

North Prong Loop

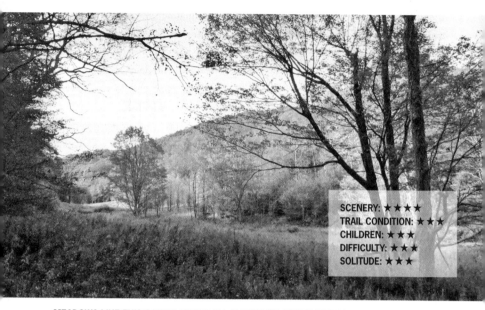

MEADOWS LIKE THIS CAN BE FOUND ALL ALONG THE NORTH PRONG LOOP.

GPS TRAILHEAD COORDINATES: N38° 42.805' W79° 34.069'

DISTANCE & CONFIGURATION: 6.7-mile loop

HIKING TIME: 3.5 hours

HIGHLIGHTS: Backcountry, meadows, some views, streams

ELEVATION: 3,960' at trailhead, 4,130' at high point, 3,500' at low point

ACCESS: No fees or permits required

MAPS: *Seneca Creek Backcountry, Monongahela National Forest;* USGS *Spruce Knob*

FACILITIES: None

WHEELCHAIR ACCESS: None

CONTACT: Cheat-Potomac Ranger District, 304-257-4488

Overview

This loop explores the south side of the Seneca Creek Backcountry. Start on the wide Allegheny Mountain Trail for some easy walking to the North Prong Trail. Descend into the valley of North Prong Big Run, passing a scenic mountain meadow before reaching Big Run. Return to Allegheny Mountain along Big Run, where a linear meadow offers ridgeline vistas. *Note:* There are numerous crossings of North Prong that can be rock-hopped in times of normal stream flow. In addition, there is one steep section at hike's end.

Route Details

Start this circuit on the Allegheny Mountain Trail, a gated forest road open for vehicular traffic only to U.S. Forest Service personnel who maintain wildlife food plots located in the Seneca Creek Backcountry. The doubletrack trailbed is mostly grassy, with occasional mucky low spots. Other small roads splinter off the main path and head to wildlife clearings, but the main track is easy to discern. A northern hardwood forest of maple, birch, and beech rises overhead, heavy with sugar maple, red maple, and striped maple. Undulate along the ridgeline at around 4,000 feet. Seneca Creek valley lies to your right and Gandy Creek valley falls away to your left. Spruce Mountain, West Virginia's highest ridge, can be seen through the trees across the Seneca Creek valley.

At 0.9 mile, enter a gap. Here, a spur road leads right to a wildlife clearing. Stay straight, climbing with the Allegheny Mountain Trail. The wide, grassy track allows you to look around and appreciate the surrounding woodlands. Undulate along the ridgeline. At 1.6 miles, at the top of a hill, a wider side road heads left to a clearing. Stay straight here, descending, still on the Allegheny Mountain Trail. Continue flirting with the 4,000-foot mark. Intersect the Tom Lick Run Trail at 2.1 miles. It leaves right to Seneca Creek. The circuit continues straight on the Allegheny Mountain Trail.

At 2.3 miles, come to the North Prong Trail amid a grassy clearing and a small coppice of planted red pine trees. Here, the Allegheny Mountain Trail leaves right, but you veer left on the doubletrack North Prong Trail, leaving the clearing behind and entering woods heavy with beech. Ascend to reach another smaller clearing at 2.7 miles. This is the loop's high point. Stay right here, quickly leave the clearing, then begin a steady descent into the North Prong Big Run watershed. Step into a large meadow at 3.2 miles. The wide glade is a mix of grasses, brush, ferns, and scattered trees through which North Prong Big Run gains steam. Curve left as the meadow slowly narrows to the valley of North Prong Big Run. Look for beaver dams on the stream.

The trailside environment changes from ridgeline to mountain stream valley. Spruce trees increase in number. North Prong comes into view. Come to a trail junction at 3.9 miles. Here, the Elza Trail crosses North Prong on an old road bridge. Stay straight, still on the North Prong Trail. Soon reach your first

North Prong Loop

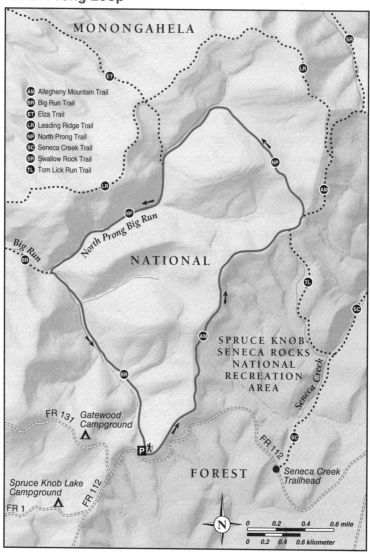

Allegheny Mountain Trail
Big Run Trail
Elza Trail
Leading Ridge Trail
North Prong Trail
Seneca Creek Trail
Swallow Rock Trail
Tom Lick Run Trail

MONONGAHELA

NATIONAL

SPRUCE KNOB-
SENECA ROCKS
NATIONAL
RECREATION
AREA

FOREST

North Prong Big Run

Big Run

FR 131   Gatewood
         Campground

Spruce Knob Lake
Campground

FR 1

FR 112

FR 112

Seneca Creek
Trailhead

Seneca Creek

0   0.2   0.4   0.6 mile
0   0.2   0.4   0.6 kilometer

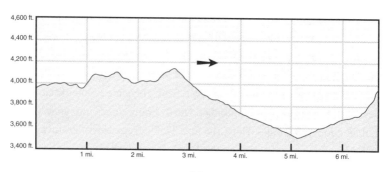

two North Prong crossings, easy rock-hops at normal water flows. The valley narrows here. Look for big moss-clad boulders and rock outcrops.

At 4.2 miles, the valley widens again as a tributary flows into North Prong. Skirt a clearing and red pine plantation at this feeder stream. Hop over the stream, continuing down North Prong. Ahead, make three crossings as the trail and stream intertwine in the slim and deep valley. As small as North Prong is, a keen eye will spot trout finning in its larger pools.

At 5.1 miles, weave through hawthorn to reach Big Run and its meadowy valley. A wooded campsite stands to your left, near the confluence of Big Run and North Prong Big Run. Turn left on the Big Run Trail, hopping North Prong one last time, then make your way up Big Run in an ever-changing composition of meadow and forest, heavy with apple and hawthorn trees. Some clearings are long and wide enough to avail ridgeline views of the surrounding mountainsides. The path stays on the north edge of the meadow, sometimes under canopy, sometimes not. Seeps flow over the trail from above. The trailbed can be rocky, muddy, and irregular, and seemingly all three at once in places. Gently ascend.

At 6.4 miles, cross the last of Big Run and its tributaries. The meadows have been left behind, and spruce finds its place among the hardwoods. Begin a solid climb that gradually steepens, eventually going straight up a north-facing hollow. Catch your breath after ending back at the Allegheny Mountain Trailhead, completing the circuit at 6.7 miles.

Nearby Attractions

Spruce Knob Lake Campground is situated in a land of superlatives: the highest campground in West Virginia, next to the highest lake in the state, and the highest point in the state. The surrounding mountains are laced with trails such as North Prong that traverse forests, fields, and streams. Campers can enjoy the cool air of the high country at drive-up campsites or walk-in tent campsites.

Directions

From the town of Seneca Rocks, head south on US 33 for 13.0 miles to Briery Gap Road. Turn right on Briery Gap Road and follow it up 2.5 miles to Forest Road (FR) 112. Turn right on FR 112 and head up 12.8 miles to the Allegheny Mountain Trailhead, which is on your right. The actual parking area is reached on a very short road to the trailhead. The Allegheny Mountain Trail starts at the back of the parking area, around the pole gate.

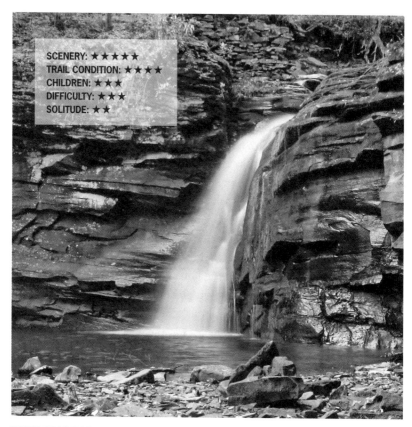

UPPER FALLS OF SENECA AND ITS PLUNGE POOL ARE A WONDER REACHED ONLY BY TRAIL.

GPS TRAILHEAD COORDINATES: N38° 42.695' W79° 32.996'

DISTANCE & CONFIGURATION: 10.2-mile out-and-back

HIKING TIME: 6 hours

HIGHLIGHTS: Other falls, Upper Falls of Seneca

ELEVATION: 3,890' at trailhead, 3,160' at low point

ACCESS: No fees or permits required

MAPS: *Seneca Creek Backcountry, Monongahela National Forest;* USGS *Spruce Knob, Whitmer*

FACILITIES: None

WHEELCHAIR ACCESS: None

CONTACT: Cheat-Potomac Ranger District, 304-257-4488

Overview

This hike could be called "Numerous Falls of Seneca," for there are many more cataracts on this hike than at the final destination, Upper Falls of Seneca. Other parts of Seneca Creek have cascades, and many tributaries of Seneca Creek have falls of their own. Throw in bucolic meadows and attractive mountain valley scenery and you have one of the finest walks in the Monongahela National Forest.

Route Details

Avid photographers will want to bring a tripod and something more than a handheld device to capture the numerous waterfalls and cascades found on this hike, highlighted by the actual Upper Falls of Seneca, found at hike's end. In addition to this 30-foot spiller, you will also find small curtain-type cataracts on Seneca Creek, slide cascades, and additional tiered drops on tributaries of Seneca Creek. Take on the challenge of not only enjoying this hike but also capturing each of these aquatic highlights situated in the trail-laden Seneca Creek Backcountry, one of the finest hiking destinations in the entire Monongahela National Forest. To that end, add extra time to photograph to your overall hike time.

Start your hike by leaving the large parking area on Forest Road (FR) 112. Pass an informative signboard, then trace the Seneca Creek Trail into the valley of Seneca Creek. The spruce-and-birch–lined path descends north. Step over Trussel Run at 0.4 mile. Seneca Creek forms where Trussel Run and Slab Camp Run meet. Just beyond this crossing look on a partly wooded meadow framed by Allegheny Mountain, dividing Seneca Creek watershed from Gandy Creek watershed to the west. Spruce Mountain rises high to the east, West Virginia's loftiest terrain.

More woods and glades lie ahead. Still other trailsides are cloaked in dark spruce thickets. Gain your first glimpses of Seneca Creek before intersecting the Tom Lick Run Trail at 0.9 mile. Stay straight on the Seneca Creek Trail as the path alternately courses through meadows, evergreens, and fern-floored hardwoods. The widening valley to your left features additional meadows and occasional beaver dams as Seneca Creek courses in serpentine fashion. Multiple feeder streams flow down from Spruce Mountain, adding volume to Seneca Creek.

Upper Falls of Seneca Creek

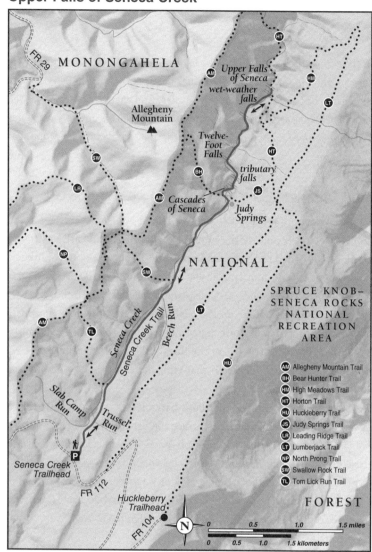

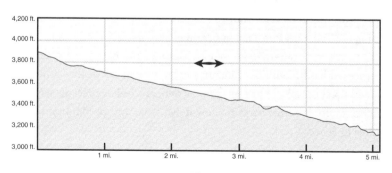

Hop over Beech Run at 2.1 miles. The trail widens below Beech Run, but the gradient remains gentle. Wind through cherry, beech, and yellow birch in a deepening and widening vale. Pass the Swallow Rock Trail at 2.3 miles. Keep following Seneca Creek downstream. At 3.0 miles, make a bridgeless crossing of Seneca Creek. This may be a ford or a rock-hop depending on the time of year. Look for bluffs and the stair-step cascades of Judy Springs across the watercourse just before arriving at the former Judy Springs Campground at 3.4 miles. This locale is still used as a campsite. A trail bridge leads across Seneca Creek to the Judy Springs Trail. To see the actual Judy Springs, cross the bridge, head right, and trace the spring outflow to a hillside rock outcrop.

To reach Upper Falls of Seneca, bypass the bridge and stay left through a field, still on the Seneca Creek Trail. Pass the Bear Hunter Trail at 3.5 miles. Bend to the right and stay along the creek as it squeezes between massive boulders. Just downstream, Seneca Creek creates two cascades—the Cascades of Seneca—as it twice pours over wide stone slabs into pools. At 3.7 miles, a little downstream from the cascades, look for a tributary waterfall entering Seneca Creek on the far side of the stream. The narrow spiller drops 40 feet altogether, first as a slender drop, then dances through rhododendron, before making a final ledge plunge to meet Seneca Creek. Next, at 3.8 miles, yet another tributary creates a fall. This one tumbles in stages about 35 feet, then filters through a gravel bar, delivering its waters to Seneca Creek.

At 3.9 miles, make an almost certain wet ford of Seneca Creek. A big trouty pool lies below the crossing, while ledge rapids sing just upstream. You are now on the right-hand bank. At 4.0 miles, look left at Twelve-Foot Falls. This tumbler drops a dozen feet into a gravel bar–bordered pool, and normally splits into chutes while pouring over ragged rock. A second fall just downstream is harder to reach, as it lies in a narrow defile.

Keep hiking, now below a mossy rock bluff, to ford Seneca Creek yet again at 4.4 miles. Keep down the valley of birch, beech, and maple, as the spruce has been left behind. You are on the left-hand bank. At 4.6 miles, squeeze past a ledge to clamber over irregular rock. Here, another fall, unnamed, drops about 10 feet over the rock strata as the strata crosses the creekbed. Bisect a small meadow at 4.9 miles. After reentering woods, look across to your right at a wet-weather falls dropping 25 feet over a ledge into Seneca Creek.

Make the final ford of Seneca Creek and meet the Horton Trail as it leaves right. Be careful here, as the ford is just above a 6-foot cascade. Continue just a bit farther and come to Upper Falls of Seneca at 5.1 miles. Get the first good look at it from the trail. Here, Seneca Creek drops 30 feet over a stone ledge bordered by a big rock overhang on the right of the fall, into a circular plunge pool. A trail leads down to the pool, where another vantage awaits. Upper Falls of Seneca is the climax of the multitude of cataracts on this hike. On your return, take time to capture images of the cavalcade of cascades on Seneca Creek.

Nearby Attractions

Spruce Knob, West Virginia's highest point at 4,861 feet, can be accessed on the drive to this hike. A short path leads to an observation tower.

Directions

From the town of Seneca Rocks, head south on US 33 for 13.0 miles to Briery Gap Road. Turn right on Briery Gap Road and follow it up 2.5 miles to FR 112. Turn right on FR 112 and head up 11.3 miles to the Seneca Creek Trailhead, on your right.

THE UPPER FALLS OF SENECA CREATES A MASSIVE PLUNGE POOL.

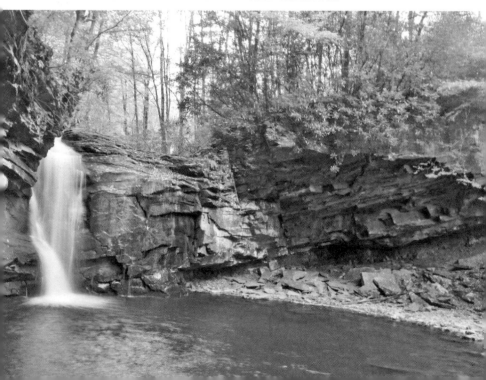

19 Spruce Knob and Huckleberry Trail

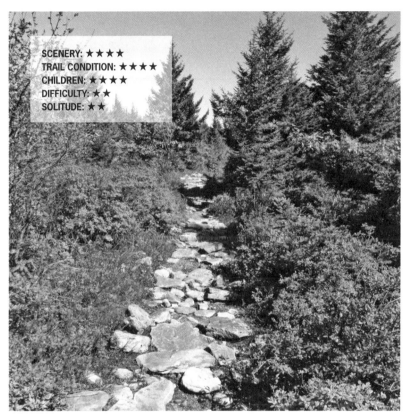

SCENERY: ★★★★
TRAIL CONDITION: ★★★★
CHILDREN: ★★★★
DIFFICULTY: ★★
SOLITUDE: ★★

THE ROCKY HUCKLEBERRY TRAIL LEADS THROUGH A MIX OF BRUSH AND SPRUCE.

GPS TRAILHEAD COORDINATES: N38° 42.695' W79° 32.996'

DISTANCE & CONFIGURATION: 0.4-mile and 4-mile out-and-back

HIKING TIME: 2.5 hours

HIGHLIGHTS: Highest point in West Virginia, talus slopes, views

ELEVATION: 4,850' at trailhead, 4,863' at high point, 4,660' at low point

ACCESS: No fees or permits required

MAPS: *Seneca Creek Backcountry, Monongahela National Forest;* USGS *Spruce Knob*

FACILITIES: Picnic area and restrooms at trailhead

WHEELCHAIR ACCESS: 0.2-mile trail to Spruce Knob

CONTACT: Cheat-Potomac Ranger District, 304-257-4488

Spruce Knob and Huckleberry Trail

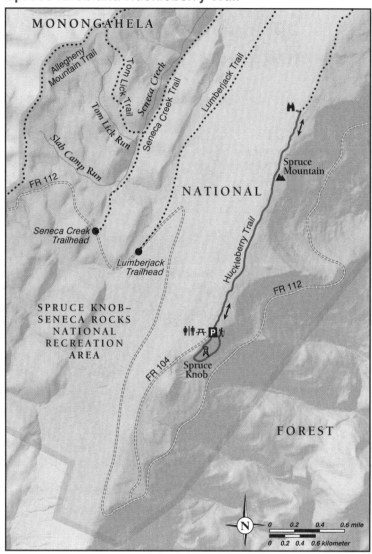

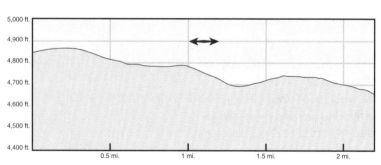

Overview

This hike takes you along a portion of the highest ridge in the state, Spruce Mountain. First, take the short walk south to the Spruce Knob Observation Tower, standing at West Virginia's highest point. Next, follow the Huckleberry Trail north along Spruce Mountain, meandering through boulder fields, spruce woods, and low-slung heath meadows to a viewpoint from a rock outcrop.

Route Details

Getting to West Virginia's highest point—Spruce Knob at 4,861 feet—is easy. All it takes is tracing a simple, wide, and nearly imperceptibly inclined trail to a squat stone tower that you can then climb to gain views of the adjacent mountains, much of which is part of the Monongahela National Forest.

There exists a whole class of people whose goal it is to visit all the highest points in every state. They are known as high pointers. Some high points can be driven to, while others require modest walks like this, such as Clingmans Dome in Tennessee or Missouri's Taum Sauk Mountain, and others require a more substantial hike, like that to Virginia's Mount Rogers or Maine's Mount Katahdin. Still others require mountaineering skills that your average hiker doesn't have or need—unless you want to climb Washington's Mount Rainier or Alaska's Denali. That being said, there are still other high points that are significant only in context to being inside the boundaries of their given state—such as Britton Hill in Florida or Ohio's Campbell Hill.

The first high pointers began making such quests in the 1930s. To this day members of high point clubs or soloists on a personal mission will be found at places like Spruce Knob, completing another quest and checking off another state.

Start this trek by doing just that. From the parking area, which features picnic sites and a restroom, head south on the Tower Trail, a wide, gentle wheelchair-accessible path. You know intellectually that the trail is going to a high point, but the grade is imperceptible. Wind-flagged spruce and stunted yellow birch rise among rock outcrops and boulder gardens. By 0.2 mile, you are at the high point, atop which sits a stone tower. Climb the steps to the tower to gain views west into the Seneca Creek Backcountry of the Monongahela National Forest, as well as ridges and mountains beyond. You can also look east toward the Old Dominion and in the other two directions if the nearby trees have been trimmed lately.

If you wish to extend your hike, the Whispering Spruce Trail makes a half-mile loop along Spruce Mountain. The interpretive path starts at the top of the tower and heads southwest along the ridgetop, then returns to the base of the tower. After making the high point, return to the trailhead at 0.4 mile. Now, take a walk along a natural-surface trail atop Spruce Mountain. Pick up the Huckleberry Trail on the north end of the parking area. A kiosk marks the path. Leave the parking area, then make a trek to your own observation point on Spruce Mountain. Enter a forest of stunted spruce trees and brush (northbound). The canopy is mostly open above the rocky path. At 0.2 mile, swing around a boulder field.

The trailbed becomes surprisingly sandy in spots. Other segments are very rocky and make for slow going. The trail alternates between dark, shady spruce thickets, where moss and spruce needles carpet the ground green and brown, contrasting with gray boulders and more open brushy areas where climate-arrested vegetation can only rise so far. Make a brief descent at 0.8 mile. However, elevation changes on this hike are only a little more than 200 feet. The woods become more thickly canopied. Level out and begin a moderate upgrade, where forest and meadow alternate. Campsites are sometimes found under thicker woods.

At mile 1.9, in a clearing, pass an upright stone marker on trail right that has 2 MI carved onto it (it was knocked over my last visit, but I put it back upright). Shortly beyond this stone marker, look for a user-created footpath leading left. Take this side trail less than 100 yards to a sloped boulder field. Fine views of the Seneca Creek Backcountry extend to your north and west. This view may not be as high as that from the observation tower, nor qualify as an official high point, but it is better earned. If you miss this first user-created path heading west to the boulder field, other trails just ahead lead left to this same outcrop.

Nearby Attractions

The Seneca Creek Trail, just a few miles distant, takes hikers to a plethora of waterfalls on a 10.2-mile round-trip through the heart of the Seneca Creek Backcountry. See Hike 18, page 96.

Directions

From the town of Seneca Rocks, head south on US 33 for 13.0 miles to Briery Gap Road. Turn right on Briery Gap Road and follow it up 2.5 miles to Forest Road (FR) 112. Turn right on FR 112 and head up 7.3 miles to FR 104. Turn right on FR 104 and follow it 2.0 miles to the Spruce Knob parking area. The Huckleberry Trail starts on the north side of the parking area, opposite the trail to the Spruce Knob Observation Tower.

20 # Laurel Fork
North Wilderness

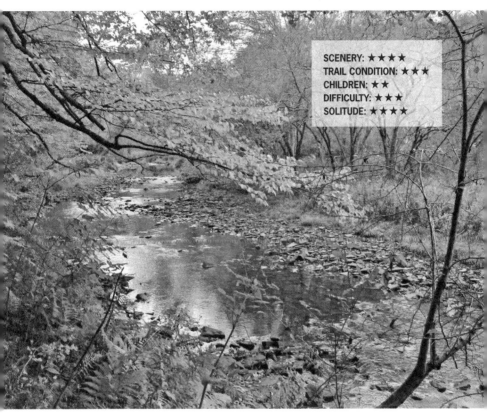

LAUREL FORK RUNS LOW IN AUTUMN.

GPS TRAILHEAD COORDINATES: N38° 44.474' W79° 41.424'

DISTANCE & CONFIGURATION: 8.6-mile out-and-back

HIKING TIME: 4.5 hours

HIGHLIGHTS: Meadows, views, wilderness

ELEVATION: 3,100' at trailhead, 2,940' at low point

ACCESS: No fees or permits required

MAPS: *Laurel Fork Wilderness, Monongahela National Forest*; USGS *Sinks of Gandy, Glady*

FACILITIES: Campground, restrooms at trailhead

WHEELCHAIR ACCESS: None

CONTACT: Greenbrier Ranger District, 304-456-3335

Laurel Fork North Wilderness

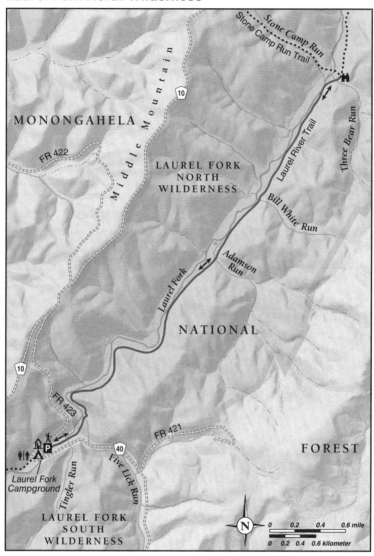

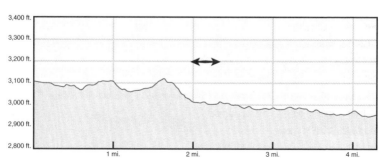

Overview

This hike takes you deep into the heart of Laurel Fork North Wilderness. Numerous trailside panoramas open of Middle Mountain and valley meadows, where Laurel Fork breaks up into numerous runs encircling large islands. The Laurel River Trail follows a mix of railroad grades and roadbeds. However, this is a federally designated wilderness; only occasional rock cairns mark your route, no signs or blazes. On the other hand, there are no major stream crossings, and elevation changes of around 200 feet ease the hiker's burden.

Route Details

When seeing it today, it is hard to imagine Laurel Fork valley was once completely logged. Originally, horses skidded trees to the waterway, then logs were floated to mills downstream. Later, a railroad through the valley made year-round logging feasible. Finally, truck-based logging moved in. However, the forest recovered, leaving us old grades now used as trails that course through the 6,055-acre Laurel Fork North Wilderness, established in 1983.

Leave the lower loop of the campground and pick up the Laurel River Trail, which departs the northern end of the loop near an information kiosk. Enter the woods on an old elevated railbed. Be watchful, as numerous camper-created errant paths may lead you astray.

Laurel Fork flows to your left yet breaks up into numerous stream braids. Cross Tingler Run at 0.1 mile. A hardwood forest of cherry, yellow birch, and occasional evergreen rises overhead. Emerge onto the first of many meadows at 0.3 mile. Rock cairns keep you on the right track, but user-created paths in these meadows can create confusion. Stay on the left side of the meadow and cross Five Lick Run at the far end of the field. Laurel Fork on your left and a steep hillside to your right pinch in the trail. Skirt a washed out segment along the edge of Laurel Fork. Views open ahead of Middle Mountain.

At 0.6 mile, Laurel River Trail bends right with the stream, comes to a field, and then diverges uphill from the river on a former logging roadbed. Climb away from the stream—the walking is pleasant through the open forest. Pass through an imperiled hemlock thicket at 1.1 miles.

Descend and return to Laurel Fork and the logging rail grade at 2.0 miles. The abandoned Middle Mountain Trail once merged here from across Laurel Fork, but it's now overgrown. Stay straight on the easy-to-trace Laurel River Trail. Laurel Fork is divided into stream braids encircling islands.

At 2.4 miles, the grade and the trail split—veer left into a clearing dotted with apple and hawthorn trees and deer paths. This is a good place to spot deer. Cross Adamson Run. Stay on the right side of the meadow and pick up the railbed once again. At 2.7 miles, tunnel through a hemlock coppice that makes day seem like dusk. A blasted-low bluff flanks your right side.

Beyond this, the valley widens. Field and forest interplay, and in clearings, Middle Mountain rises into view to your left. Laurel Fork forms a complicated drainage made more perplexing by beaver dams. At 3.1 miles, step over Bill White Run and immediately climb into a small clearing with a rock cairn. Stay straight on the logging road grade. Look below for the old rail grade.

Return to the railroad grade along Laurel Fork. A massive meadow opens to your left as the valley floor widens. At 4.2 miles, the trail curves right. Cross Three Bear Run. By 4.3 miles, the trail reaches a junction marked with a big rock cairn. To your left, the Stone Camp Run Trail crosses a meadow and Laurel Fork, then heads 1.5 miles up Middle Mountain to Forest Road (FR) 14. The Laurel River Trail continues down the valley. This intersection is your destination. You can capture great views of Middle Mountain across in the meadow and relax in the woods of Three Bear Run, or view some fine pools just downstream on Laurel Fork. Unwind and take in some wilderness before heading back.

Nearby Attractions

The hike starts at Laurel Fork Campground, open during the warm season and a good base camp to explore both Laurel Fork North Wilderness and Laurel Fork South Wilderness. Sixteen campsites are spread over two loops in a partly wooded flat alongside Laurel Fork. Each campsite has a table, lantern holder, and fire ring. Vault toilets serve the two loops. Bring your own water.

Directions

From Elkins, drive east on US 33 for 12.6 miles over Alpena Gap to the hamlet of Alpena. Turn right on County Road (CR) 27 (Glady Road), just across from the Alpine Motel. Follow CR 27 for 9.2 miles to Glady. Turn left on Middle Mountain Road (FR 422) and drive 4.6 miles to FR 14. Turn right on FR 14 and drive south 0.3 mile to FR 423. Turn left on FR 423 and drive 1.5 miles down to Laurel Fork Campground. Cross the bridge over Laurel Fork, then turn left into the lower loop. Pick up the Laurel River Trail at the north end of the loop, near a signboard and campsite 13.

Camp Five Run Loop

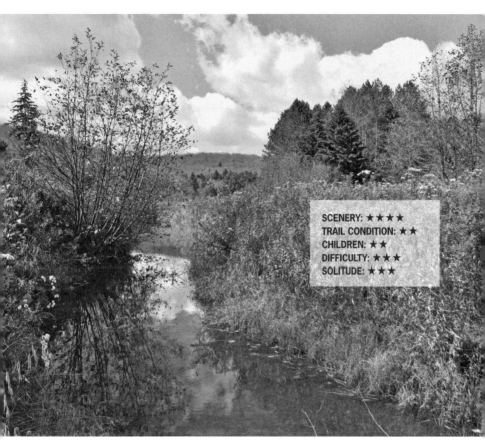

SCENERY: ★ ★ ★ ★
TRAIL CONDITION: ★ ★
CHILDREN: ★ ★
DIFFICULTY: ★ ★ ★
SOLITUDE: ★ ★ ★

UPPER LAUREL FORK FLOWS SLOWLY IN ITS BEAVER-DAMMED UPPER REACHES.

GPS TRAILHEAD COORDINATES: N38° 41.267' W79° 44.126'

DISTANCE & CONFIGURATION: 6.4-mile loop

HIKING TIME: 3.5 hours

HIGHLIGHTS: Meadows and woods, mountain views, wildlife

ELEVATION: 3,620' at trailhead, 3,850' at high point, 3,370' at low point

ACCESS: No fees or permits required

MAPS: *Laurel Fork Wilderness, Monongahela National Forest*; USGS *Sinks of Gandy*

FACILITIES: National forest rental cabins, pump well near trailhead

WHEELCHAIR ACCESS: None

CONTACT: Greenbrier Ranger District, 304-456-3335

Camp Five Run Loop

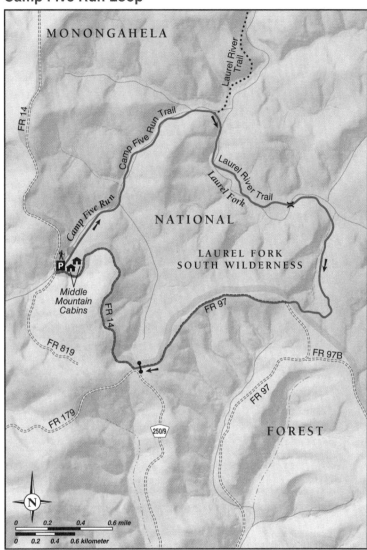

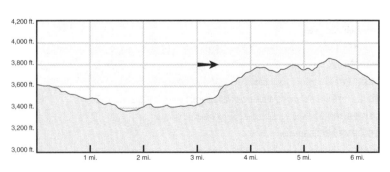

Overview

This loop is a treat for the eyes while exploring Laurel Fork South Wilderness. Start your hike near the historic Middle Mountain Cabins, then descend along Camp Five Run, passing numerous meadows along the way. Turn up Laurel Fork, then enter a huge meadow with great valley and mountain panoramas. Climb to the high country and an experimental forest area with more views. Close the loop with a walk along a quiet forest road. Be advised: portions of the trails along this circuit can be hard to follow, but with a little reckoning—and a GPS—you should have no problem.

Route Details

Leave the parking area on Forest Road (FR) 14 and walk down gravel FR 819 a short distance to pass the Middle Mountain Cabins on your right. Keep straight on the Camp Five Run Trail—a former railroad bed—as it passes a dammed pond, then enters Laurel Fork South Wilderness at 0.2 mile. Keep following the grade downhill through a mix of spruce and northern hardwoods. Rock-hop Camp Five Run at 0.6 mile.

Step across Camp Five Run twice in succession at 0.7 mile, then enter a linear field. Make a fourth crossing at 0.9 mile. You are now on the right bank of Camp Five Run. The trail soon climbs away from the grade and follows a foot trail, only to regain the railroad grade. Leave the railroad grade a second time for good at 1.2 miles, where the trail splits off to the right. A large meadow stretches to your left.

The footpath remains in woods as the meadow to your left increases in size. At 1.6 miles, reach a wooden post indicating the intersection with the Laurel River Trail/Forest Trail #306. This is the end of the Camp Five Run Trail. Veer right and join the Laurel River Trail, cutting through red pine and spruce woodland, and then pick up a railbed. Field, fern, and forest mix and meld, with much evidence of beavers: still ponds and chewed-down trees. At 1.8 miles, make a bridgeless crossing of Laurel Fork, ensconced in alder thickets. Reenter the woods, then watch for the trail splitting left, still heading upstream along another roadbed. Follow this grassy path, ignoring other trails dropping down to Laurel Fork at 2.0 miles. One of these errant trails has a capped well on it. Views open to the southwest.

At 2.1 miles, look for rock cairns in a tricky section just before crossing a wet, grassy streambed. On the far side of the streambed is a red pine plantation.

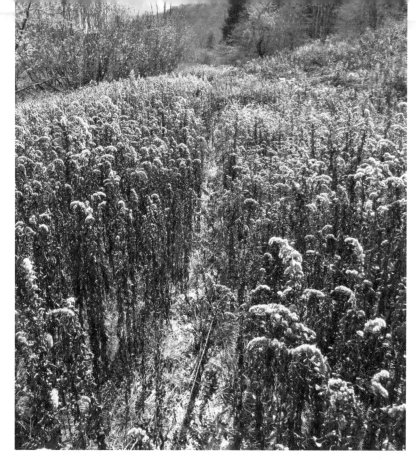

AUTUMN-TINGED BRUSH LINES THE WILDERNESS PATH.

Turn right toward Laurel Fork at a cairn, then cross the mushy streambed, joining a roadbed. Follow this grassy roadbed into the pine plantation.

The wide road winds beneath the needle-carpeted woods, then enters a big meadow and comes to cross Laurel Fork at 2.6 miles. Beavers have been historically active in this area, damming Laurel Fork. Therefore, you may have a wet crossing. Turn left once across Laurel Fork, following a roadbed upstream along the right side of the meadow. Expansive valley and ridge panoramas make this a highlight of the trip, despite navigational challenges.

The trail, passing through mostly open terrain, becomes somewhat wooded again as it crosses an unnamed tributary coming in from your right at 3.0 miles. Just after this crossing, the trail turns up and to your right (south) away from the meadow to parallel the tributary you just crossed. Leave the meadow and ascend. The forest canopy closes overhead. Spruce trees increase in number.

At 3.6 miles, the trail swings right around the head of a hollow and continues to climb. Come to trail signs and gated FR 97 at 3.9 miles. Turn right on the gravel forest road. Along this road, closed to the public except for certain hunting seasons, is an ongoing tree-farming experiment. The science of tree farming is known as silviculture.

Views to the south and southwest open up as you travel the hardwood-clad ridge. Reach a gate where signs explain the tree experiments and FR 14 at 5.1 miles. You are now 3,760 feet high. Turn right on FR 14 and head north, climbing past a knob to reach a high point at 5.5 miles. It is all downhill from here. Reach the gravel road of the Middle Mountain Cabins (FR 819), completing your loop at 6.4 miles.

Nearby Attractions

This hike passes by the Middle Mountain Cabins, three rustic wooden structures set in a small clearing in a remote section of the Monongahela National Forest. The cabins, available for rental from April through November, sleep 8–10 people. Cabin users share a pump well and vault toilets. Built in 1931 and 1939 for Monongahela National Forest personnel, they have since been converted for recreational use by forest visitors. The cabins, listed on the National Register of Historic Places, can be reserved online at recreation.gov.

Directions

From Elkins, drive east on US 33 for 12.6 miles over Alpena Gap to the hamlet of Alpena. Turn right on County Road (CR) 27 (Glady Road), just across from the Alpine Motel. Follow CR 27 for 9.2 miles to Glady. Turn left on Middle Mountain Road (FR 422) and drive 4.6 miles to FR 14. Turn right on FR 14 and follow it south 4.5 miles to the Middle Mountain Cabins, on your left. Park at the intersection of FR 14 and the road to Middle Mountain Cabins, FR 819, taking care not to block any roads.

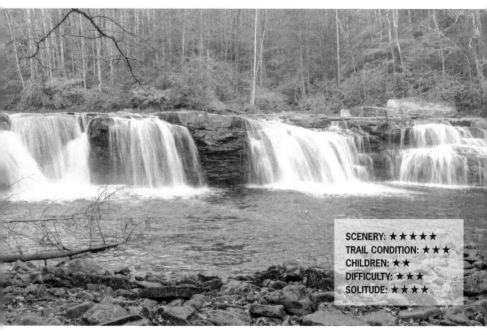

HIGH FALLS RUSHES OVER ITS STONE FACE.

SCENERY: ★★★★★
TRAIL CONDITION: ★★★
CHILDREN: ★★
DIFFICULTY: ★★★
SOLITUDE: ★★★★

GPS TRAILHEAD COORDINATES: N38° 44.997' W79° 45.153'

DISTANCE & CONFIGURATION: 7.6-mile out-and-back

HIKING TIME: 4 hours

HIGHLIGHTS: High Falls, meadows, Red Run Falls

ELEVATION: 3,020' at trailhead, 3,630' at high point

ACCESS: No fees or permits required

MAPS: *Monongahela National Forest;* USGS *Beverly East*

FACILITIES: None

WHEELCHAIR ACCESS: None

CONTACT: Greenbrier Ranger District, 304-456-3335

Overview

This hike takes you to a powerful and scenic falls, as well as a lesser cascade, in addition to climbing over a mountain and traversing a mountain clearing. Leave the West Fork Glady Fork valley and surmount Shavers Mountain. Descend

Shavers Mountain to big Shavers Fork. There, follow a little-used railroad track past Red Run Falls and continue downstream along Shavers Fork to brawny High Falls, which makes a river-wide drop.

Route Details

Though you do have specific highlights on this hike—namely High Falls—the trek takes you through numerous alluring sights, from the crossing of Glady Fork, to the meadow of the former community of Beulah, to the spruce-clad crest of Shavers Mountain, to noisy Red Run Falls. So expect to see beauty throughout your adventure.

Leave Forest Road (FR) 44 on the High Falls Trail. Quickly descend to an old roadbed, heading left (southwest). Parallel FR 44, then veer right at 0.1 mile, entering a partially wooded meadow. Reach West Fork Glady Fork at 0.2 mile. Cross the smallish, clear mountain stream on a wooden footbridge, then pass through the remains of a wooden gate. Wind through more meadows broken with hawthorn trees and come to the West Fork Trail and the former commu nity of Beulah at 0.4 mile. Remains of wooden fences are scattered in the locale where cattle once grazed, where pastures are slowly morphing to woodland, where houses once stood but are now reverting to wilds again.

Stay straight on the High Falls Trail, now running in conjunction with West Virginia's master path, the Allegheny Trail. Ascend through meadowland. Shavers Mountain looms ahead. Make sure to look back toward Little Beech Mountain.

Rise into woods and switchback up the southwest slope of Shavers Moun tain on a rocky singletrack path. Keep climbing through maple-beech woods, bisecting a logging road at 1.2 miles. Continue ascending to arrive at a gap with a campsite, then a trail junction at 1.6 miles, now atop Shavers Mountain. To your left the Allegheny Trail runs south along the crest of Shavers Mountain toward Wildell trail shelter. Keep straight on the High Falls Trail. This is the literal high point of the hike. You now move into the Shavers Fork valley.

Step over a spring, then swing through an evergreen forest littered with mossy rocks. Intersect an obvious grassy lane at 1.9 miles. Turn right and fol low the road. The walking is easy. At 2.0 miles, dive left into the woods at a signed turn. Back on singletrack trail, the path descends the northwest slope of Shavers Mountain via several switchbacks on a rock-lined footpath. Step over intermittent streambeds, traverse rock fields, and pick through small rhodo dendron groves. The going is slow in this stony section.

High Falls

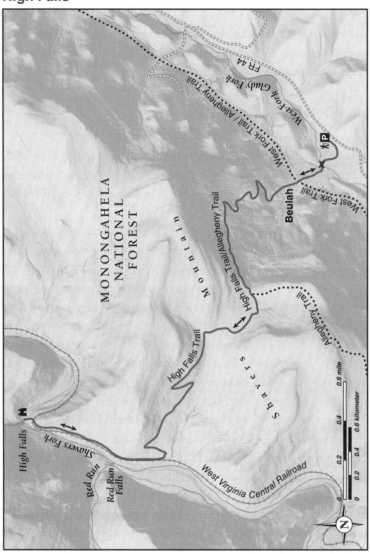

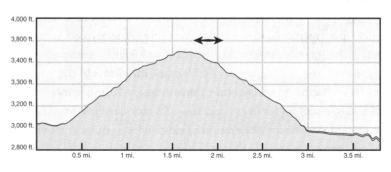

Shavers Fork soon becomes audible below. The trailside boulders are bigger the closer you get to the river. Reach the former West Virginia Central Railroad at 3.0 miles. The ties and tracks are still here, though the track is only sparingly used as an excursion train route. Turn right at the railroad tracks and follow parallel to them downstream with Shavers Fork to your left. In other spots, small culverts and narrow spots eliminate the parallel path and you have to walk the tracks. Stay off the tracks as much as possible. Cheat Mountain rises to your left, while Shavers Fork crashes down below, then quiets in alternating pools. More white rapids rumble ahead.

Spur trails lead down to Shavers Fork. At 3.3 miles, one spur leads down to a gravel bar where you can gaze across Shavers Fork at Red Run Falls. The cataract spills about 10 feet over a rock ledge into a pool. Most trail travelers pass by this spiller. Continue down the tracks, curving right just before reaching High Falls at 3.8 miles. Here, picnic tables, restrooms, and a wooden shelter stand by the tracks, while wooden steps lead to the falls and to multiple views.

Shavers Fork curves in a horseshoe of more than 100 feet in length and drops about 16 feet into a deep hole. Enjoy views of the falls from the upper observation deck, the open-rock slabs above the falls, as well as from the rock bar below this wonder of the Monongahela National Forest. The falls really roars when the water is up.

Nearby Attractions

The West Fork Trail, which you cross on this hike, is a 22-mile rail-trail that extends roughly from Glady to Durbin through the Monongahela National Forest. It offers a great opportunity for casual bicyclers and hikers to enjoy a deep mountain valley without extensive effort. The West Fork Trail has multiple accesses, making trips of varied lengths easy.

Directions

From Elkins, drive east on US 33 for 12.6 miles over Alpena Gap to the hamlet of Alpena. Turn right on County Road (CR) 27 (Glady Road), just across from the Alpine Motel. Follow CR 27 for 9.2 miles to Glady. Turn left on Middle Mountain Road (CR 22) and follow it for 0.2 mile to Glady-Durbin Road (FR 44). Turn right on FR 44, which soon turns to gravel. Keep on FR 44 for 3.9 miles to the High Falls Trail, which starts on your right. The roadside parking is a little before you reach the sign for High Falls Trail.

23 Shavers Mountain via Johns Camp Run

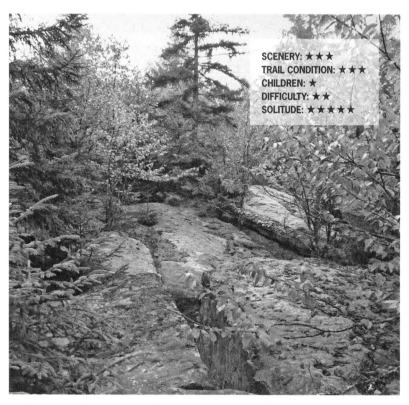

SCENERY: ★★★
TRAIL CONDITION: ★★★
CHILDREN: ★
DIFFICULTY: ★★
SOLITUDE: ★★★★★

SCRAMBLING THROUGH THIS BOULDER GARDEN ADDS A TWIST TO THIS HIKE.

GPS TRAILHEAD COORDINATES: N38° 40.105' W79° 49.755'

DISTANCE & CONFIGURATION: 4.8-mile out-and-back

HIKING TIME: 3 hours

HIGHLIGHTS: Allegheny Trail, solitude, trail shelter, views

ELEVATION: 3,620' at trailhead, 4,180' at high point

ACCESS: No fees or permits required

MAPS: *Monongahela National Forest;* USGS *Wildell*

FACILITIES: None

WHEELCHAIR ACCESS: None

CONTACT: Greenbrier Ranger District, 304-456-3335

Overview

This hike takes you through a lesser-traveled area of the national forest. Take the Johns Camp Run Trail to the Allegheny Trail and a trail shelter. Head north on the Allegheny Trail on Shavers Mountain to a knob and boulder outcrop, where a rock scramble leads to views of the surrounding mountains. This rock scramble over massive boulders is not suitable for children.

Route Details

You will drive by the Gaudineer Scenic Area Trailhead—the half-mile hike through old-growth spruce and birch—on the way to this hike. Therefore, it may be tempting to stop and do the half-mile walk before you head up Johns Camp Run, where a remote boulder garden and a view await. No matter whether you walk the old-growth Gaud ineer Scenic Area forest first or second, just walk it. After all, the 50 acres of virgin spruce forest, with trees exceeding 3 feet in diameter, are a National Natural Landmark.

For the Shavers Mountain hike via Johns Camp Run, leave the small parking area at the end of primitive Forest Road (FR) 317 on the Johns Camp Run Trail. Pass an earthen vehicle barricade. The grassy path is lined with young spruce amid yellow birch, cherry, and beech towering over spreading ferns. The climb is moderate on the singletrack path overlain on a long-closed forest road. Small streams cross the trail but pose no barriers, as they are all easy step-overs. Johns Camp Run, to your left, chatters its way downstream to meet Shavers Fork.

Work your way through some mucky areas. At 0.5 mile, the path abruptly leaves the grade right and winds upward through the woods as a foot trail. Step over a spring branch at 0.7 mile, then reach a trail intersection at 0.8 mile. Here, the Johns Camp Run Trail meets West Virginia's master path—the 330-mile Allegheny Trail, blazed in its familiar yellow rectangles. The Johns Camp Run trail shelter is located at this intersection. Here in a gap on Shavers Mountain, the three-sided, open-fronted Adirondack shelter harbors overnight campers walking the Allegheny Trail. The spring branch you crossed at 0.7 mile flows by the wooden structure. A fire ring sits in front of the refuge.

Unlike shelters on the Appalachian Trail, this one is seldom used and you are almost guaranteed solitude when spending the night here. I have stayed here twice and had it both times to myself. Not only that, but you will likely

Shavers Mountain via Johns Camp Run

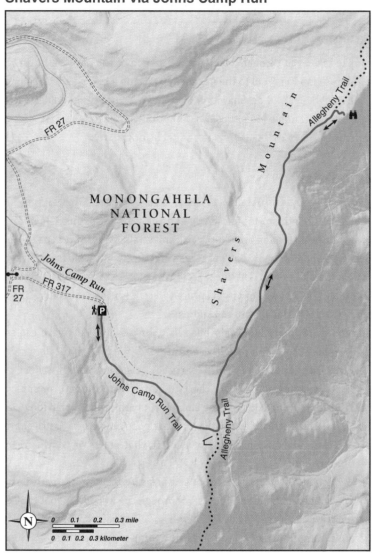

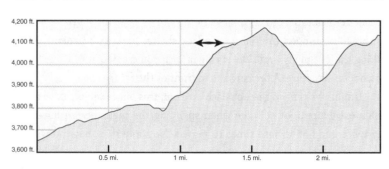

have this entire hike to yourself. Remoteness and seclusion are two highlights of this adventure.

Turn left (north) on the Allegheny Trail, following the yellow blazes toward the Wildell shelter. Climb out of the gap. Hardwoods and evergreens crowd the lightly used section of the Allegheny Trail. Top out at 1.6 miles, reaching the high point of the hike, hovering just below 4,200 feet amid spruce. You are on the right-hand side of the ridge. Obscured views of the Greenbrier River valley, Middle Mountain, and the Alleghenies stretch beyond.

Continue on the Allegheny Trail, descending ferny, mossy, rock-strewn hardwoods to reach a gap at 2.0 miles. To your right, water flows to the West Fork Greenbrier River then south to the New River, while water to your left flows into Shavers Fork then north to the Cheat River. Both part of the Ohio River watershed, they take wildly different routes to diffuse their waters. Ascend the nose of the ridge to another knob rising to your right. By 2.3 miles, big mossy boulders litter the forested terrain.

Here, look for the highest outcrop of boulders off to your right, and begin to climb up them to a high point. Faint trails from a few previous explorers may help guide the way. This high point, a couple hundred feet distant, is not very obvious from the trail. Be very careful while scrambling, as there are 10- to 15-foot crevasses between some of these cabin-size boulders. From the highest boulder, views can be had of Cheat Mountain to your west. More scrambling will avail some views back to the east. This rock jumble is a fun place to explore, finding more vistas and small rock shelters of your own. One thing you will find for sure is solitude.

After backtracking to the trailhead, be sure to walk among the giants in the Gaudineer Scenic Area. The exemplary red spruce and hardwood are a product of a mistake in pre–Civil War surveying and logging. The surveyors forgot to factor in true north as opposed to magnetic north, which is 4 degrees off from true north at this longitude. Later, someone claimed the mismeasured slice of land, resulting in the narrow, 900-acre parcel being spared the logger's axe. It was later purchased by the U.S. Forest Service and now stands as an outstanding intact plant community worth a walk to visit.

Nearby Attractions

The Gaudineer Scenic Area not only has a half-mile nature trail that winds through old-growth spruce and northern hardwoods, but you can also dine at the designated picnic area on Shavers Mountain.

Directions

From the Greenbrier Ranger Station in Bartow, head north on US 250 for 7.5 miles to FR 27 and a sign for Gaudineer Scenic Area. Turn right on FR 27 and follow it 6.2 miles to primitive FR 317 (along the way you will first pass the left turn to Gaudineer Picnic Area, then drive by the Gaudineer Scenic Area Trailhead on your right). Turn right on FR 317 and follow it 0.4 mile to a dead end at the Johns Camp Run Trailhead.

EAST FORK GREENBRIER RIVER FLOWS PAST A COLORFUL MOUNTAINSIDE.

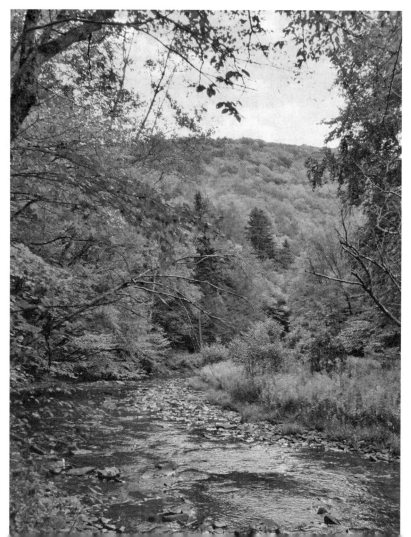

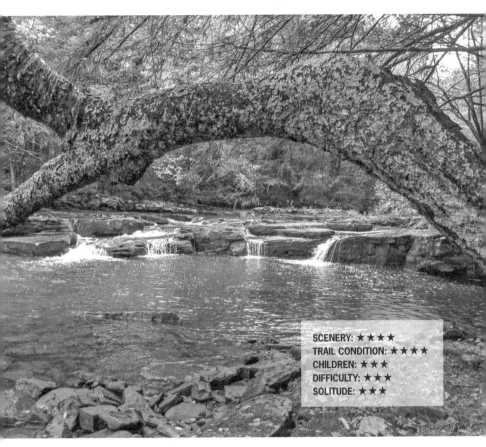

THESE HORSESHOE-SHAPED FALLS CREATE A FINE SUMMERTIME SWIMMING HOLE.

SCENERY: ★★★★
TRAIL CONDITION: ★★★★
CHILDREN: ★★★
DIFFICULTY: ★★★
SOLITUDE: ★★★

GPS TRAILHEAD COORDINATES: N38° 34.754' W79° 42.214'

DISTANCE & CONFIGURATION: 8-mile out-and-back

HIKING TIME: 4.5 hours

HIGHLIGHTS: Cascades, river valley, varied environments

ELEVATION: 3,005' at trailhead, 3,260' at high point

ACCESS: No fees or permits required

MAPS: *Monongahela National Forest;* USGS *Thornwood*

FACILITIES: Campground, restrooms at trailhead

WHEELCHAIR ACCESS: None

CONTACT: Greenbrier Ranger District, 304-456-3335

East Fork Greenbrier Hike

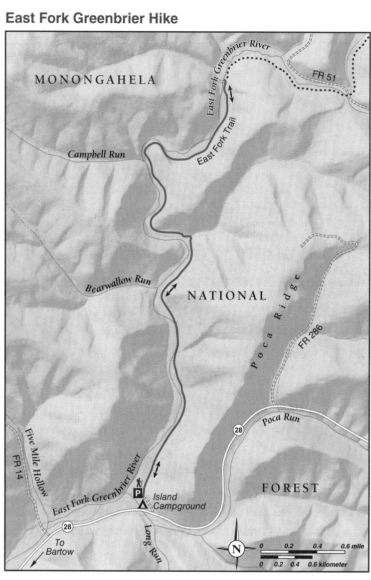

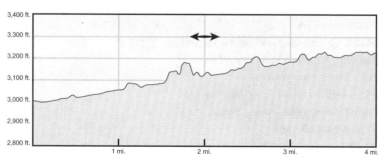

Overview

This hike leads along the headwaters of one of West Virginia's most famed rivers—the Greenbrier. Walk the valley of East Fork of the Greenbrier River through forests, meadows, and plantings of red spruce to a small waterfall, which makes a good destination and turnaround point. This valley hike can be done any time of year, since it stays on the right bank of the stream its entire length, using old roads, grades, and trails, and thus has no fords. Spring hikers will be rewarded with wildflowers, while summertime finds anglers and swimmers trailside. Fall colors are especially attractive here, and the cascades at hike's end will exude different faces in every season.

Route Details

Leave Island Campground northbound on the doubletrack East Fork Trail, working around vehicle-blocking boulders. Do not walk west over old wooden bridges from the campground turnaround or south toward campsite 12. Pass a signboard, then head up the East Fork of the Greenbrier River valley on a gentle grade beneath a deciduous forest with pockets of evergreens. The East Fork flows to your left in a series of braids with the main channel across the flat from the trail. Small glades and islands form an intertwined wetland, reworked to improve trout habitat. Poca Ridge rises to your right.

The walking is easy and nearly level. The hike as a whole rises only 260 feet over 4.0 miles, infinitesimal by West Virginia mountain standards, but does go up and down along the right bank of the river as the terrain requires. Come alongside East Fork at 0.4 mile. Look down on the mountain rill. This crystalline headwater stream holds wary trout in its pools. These fish scatter upon your passing. The East Fork Trail becomes hemmed in by East Fork to your left and Poca Ridge to your right. The river and trail soon separate.

At 0.7 mile, step over a braid of the stream, joining an island. Quickly veer right, recrossing the braid. Continue northbound under birch and maple. The trail and stream continue to play tag. Return to the river at 1.0 mile, then climb a bluff above the East Fork, separating from the old logging grade, now on singletrack path. Your elevated position allows good views into the East Fork. Pass above a river-wide ledge cascade at 1.2 miles. Upstream, the East Fork descends over flat rock slabs into sizable pools.

At 1.4 miles, drop back to the river, then open into a big meadow interspersed with hawthorn and apple trees. You can see the ridges surrounding Bearwallow Run, entering the East Fork across the meadow. Stay on the right edge of the meadow. Toward the end of the clearing, as the river curves to the right, the trail curves up the hillside to your right, joining an old roadbed. At 1.9 miles, look below for a huge pool on East Fork.

Step over a side stream coming in from your right at 2.0 miles, then drop once again to the East Fork. The streamside flat is mostly covered in trees, with some open areas grown up in ferns, which turn gold in early fall. Look for signs of beaver activity here, such as chewed-down trees, stripped limbs, and old dams. At 2.3 miles, toward the end of the flat, the trail again jogs right onto the hillside, climbing to avoid fords. Work along the ridge and drop to the valley floor again at 2.7 miles, ending up in a streamside spruce thicket. Enjoy walking through the soft-floored fairy tale forest.

LOOKING DOWN ON EAST FORK FROM WHERE THE TRAIL RISES TO AVOID A FORD.

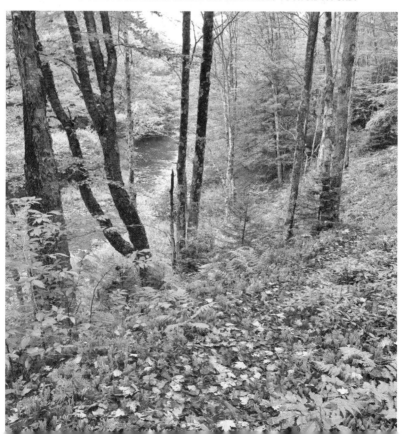

At 2.9 miles, Campbell Run enters across the river, while the East Fork and the East Fork Trail make a 180-degree bend to the right. The evergreen-rich flat, with brown needle-covered bottoms, ends at mile 3.1 as the trail is pinched in by the watercourse and hillside. Once again, the trail climbs away from the floodplain, now in yellow birch woodland. Achieve the river bottom at 3.6 miles. Notice East Fork is smaller upstream of Campbell Run. As the pattern goes, climb again up the hillside, then drop into another spruce thicket at 3.5 miles. Continue upstream.

Just as you leave the river bottom again, at 4.0 miles on your left, a waterfall drops on the East Fork. A stone ledge forms a horseshoe, spilling into a deep pool suitable for swimming. The cataract drops about 5 feet on the far right, where the circular, deep pool lies. The middle of the falls is a ledge broken by rapids, and the far left is a mix of ledges and rapids. Water flow rates can change this composition. There is a lightly used campsite here, and it is easy to work your way downstream to the base of the pool. The falls and pool create a worthy destination. Note that upstream East Fork makes a few more rapids and pools worth visiting. If you want to see the additional pools and cascades, stay along the creek and not on the official hiking trail.

Nearby Attractions

Island Campground, open April through November, is located at the trailhead and is popular with anglers fishing East Fork. Ten smallish auto-accessible, first come, first served campsites and two walk-in tent sites are there to enjoy, between WV 28 and East Fork. Each campsite has a table, lantern holder, and fire ring. Vault toilets serve the camping area. Bring your own water.

Directions

From the Monongahela National Forest ranger station in the town of Bartow on US 250, take US 250 south/WV 28 north 2.2 miles, then veer left on WV 28 (US 250 veers right). Follow WV 28 for 2.7 more miles, then turn left into Island Campground. Drive to the auto turnaround at the rear of the campground. Park there, and the East Fork Trail leaves right, north from the turnaround.

Greater Cranberry Wilderness Area

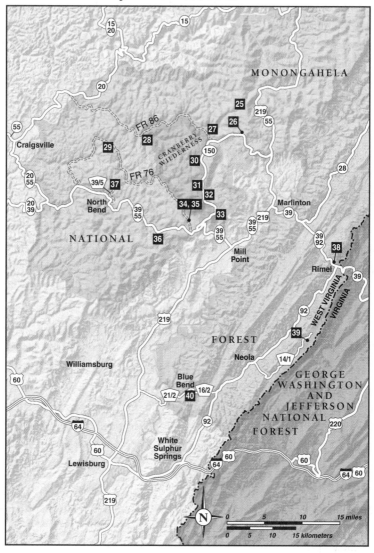

Greater Cranberry
Wilderness Area

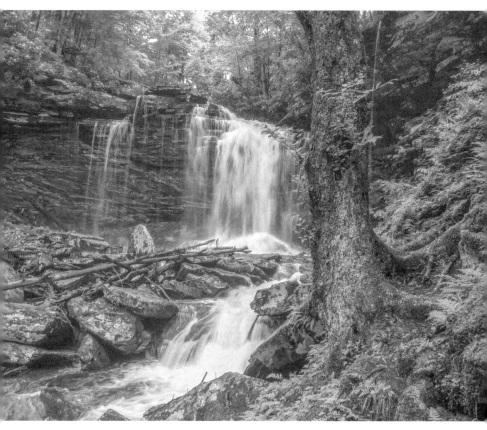

MIDDLE FALLS IS ONE OF THE FAMED FALLS OF HILLS CREEK. *(See Hike 36, page 178.)*

25 **Bear Pen Ridge Loop**

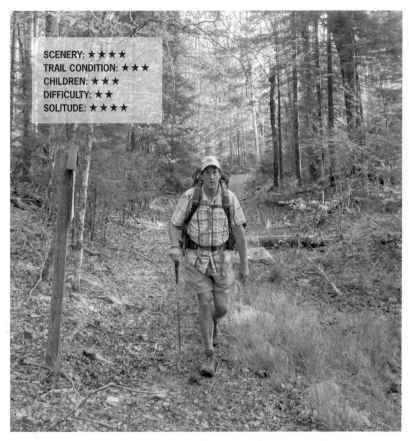

AUTHOR IN THE MIDST OF AN OVERNIGHT BACKPACK ON THE BEAR PEN RIDGE LOOP

GPS TRAILHEAD COORDINATES: N38° 23.569' W80° 09.532'

DISTANCE & CONFIGURATION: 7.3-mile loop

HIKING TIME: 3.3 hours

HIGHLIGHTS: Solitude, trail shelters

ELEVATION: 4,304' at trailhead, 3,859' at low point

ACCESS: No fees or permits required

MAPS: *Tea Creek Area Hiking Trails, Monongahela National Forest;* USGS *Sharp Knob, Woodrow*

FACILITIES: None

WHEELCHAIR ACCESS: None

CONTACT: Marlinton–White Sulphur Ranger District, 304-799-4334

Overview

This circuit offers a highland hike cloaked in solitude, with everywhere-you-look beauty, set in the underused Tea Creek Backcountry. Start at 4,300 feet, then descend along upper Tea Creek, passing a trail shelter. Hike along singing Tea Creek before rising along seldom-hiked Bear Pen Ridge Trail, coming to a second trail shelter. Return along the rim of Gauley Mountain on an easy track, as the ridgecrest slopes steeply below.

Route Details

After extensively hiking the Monongahela National Forest for three-plus decades, I fail to understand why the Tea Creek Backcountry isn't more popular. Located just north of revered and busy Cranberry Wilderness, the untamed Tea Creek Backcountry features 44 miles of hiking trails. Elevations range from 3,000 feet to over 4,500 feet. The mostly gentle pathways—well marked and signed— follow old railroad logging grades, making for foot-friendly hiking. Solitude seekers should head here during busy times. I've done this very loop on a warm weather Saturday and didn't see another hiker. You may see a few mountain bikers.

This particular circuit, with a little over 1,000 feet of elevation gain/loss, explores uppermost Tea Creek and presents two backcountry trail shelters that beg an overnight campout. And the first shelter is less than a mile distant from the trailhead, making an easy trek with camping gear. Head south on the Tea Creek Trail, tracing a wide, level track, southbound. Spruce dominates overhead and is complemented by beech, maple, and scattered yellow birch. To your right a wall of stone evinces former mining activity along this part of Gauley Mountain. Pass a small, clear pond, rimmed in grass, at 0.1 mile.

The southbound trail gently curves around a knob to your right, then runs headlong into the upper Tea Creek shelter, set in a tiny clearing, at 0.7 mile. The three-sided wooden refuge is open in the front. A picnic table and fire ring fulfill the picture. Water can be had from the headwaters of Tea Creek, just beyond the shelter. Tea Creek Trail descends sharply behind the shelter along a streamlet, then joins an old railroad grade, to meet the Tea Creek–Gauley Connector, a short path, at 1.0 mile. Note the metal trail maps located at junctions, adding navigational ease. Stay right with the Tea Creek Trail on the grade, making a switchback at 1.4 miles, then crossing Tea Creek at 1.7 miles. The downgrade parallels the tannin-colored stream as it babbles west among rocks and fallen timber. Beavers are at work here, and you will undoubtedly see the stick dams

Bear Pen Ridge Loop

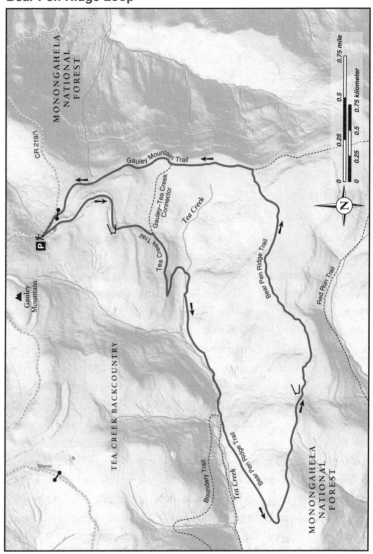

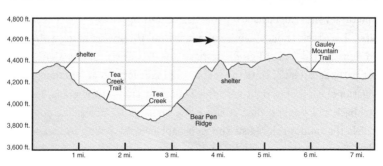

with serene pools behind them. Drop below 4,000 feet. Hardwoods become more numerous. Small branches trickle down Bear Pen Ridge. At 2.2 miles, the trail has been rerouted around a washout. Soon return to the grade and reach an old logging camp at 2.4 miles. Scan the artificial flat for metal relics.

Cross Tea Creek twice in rapid succession, then at 2.6 miles reach a three-way intersection. Stay left on Bear Pen Ridge Trail as the Boundary Trail crosses Tea Creek and the Tea Creek Trail keeps downstream. Bear Pen Ridge Trail ascends the mountainside and makes an abrupt turn east, still climbing. Ramble over a pair of rocky knobs to reach a little-used, south-facing trail shelter in a gap at 4.2 miles. A spring down a draw to the south provides water. I've overnighted here and give it a hearty recommendation.

Bear Pen Ridge Trail continues easterly along the ridge among tightly knit mountain laurel and rhododendron. The trail is either level or has a slight uptick. Flat segments bring the inevitable bogs, around which the trail is sometimes routed. Top out at 5.6 miles. The path dives off the east face of Gauley Mountain, reaching a junction at 5.8 miles. Here, head left on the Gauley Mountain Trail, a wide easy track perched on the rim of the ridge. Obscured views can be had down to Old Field Fork and across to Buzzard Mountain.

Come near an open meadow at 6.2 miles. Pass the other end of the Tea Creek–Gauley Connector at 6.3 miles. Return to the rim of the mountain and keep northbound. Elevated berms make the walking easy. Stay on the rim, passing big gray boulders and small spring branches. Pop out onto County Road (CR) 219/1 at a gate at 7.2 miles. From here, turn left and walk up the gravel track 0.1 mile, returning to the trailhead and completing the circuit.

Nearby Attractions

Tea Creek Campground is located at the lower, western part of the Tea Creek Backcountry and offers rustic, serene camping along lower Tea Creek, with access to the nearby big Williams River.

Directions

From Marlinton, drive north on US 219 for 14.4 miles to turn left onto CR 219/1 (Mine Road; you'll see a sign for "Gauley Base" trails). Follow CR 219/1 for 3.6 miles, passing the Gauley Mountain Trail just before reaching the trailhead parking on your left.

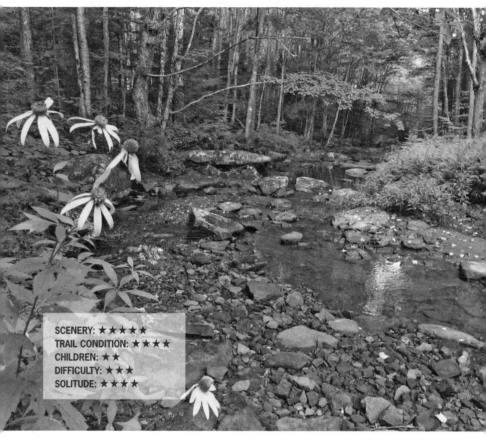

SCENERY: ★★★★★
TRAIL CONDITION: ★★★★
CHILDREN: ★★
DIFFICULTY: ★★★
SOLITUDE: ★★★★

WILDFLOWERS GRACE THE CREEK CROSSING ON RIGHT FORK.

GPS TRAILHEAD COORDINATES: N38° 20.513' W80° 9.441'

DISTANCE & CONFIGURATION: 7.2-mile loop

HIKING TIME: 4 hours

HIGHLIGHTS: Meadows, some views, well-marked trail system

ELEVATION: 4,260' at trailhead, 4,440' at high point, 3,930' at low point

ACCESS: No fees or permits required

MAPS: *Tea Creek Area Hiking Trails, Monongahela National Forest;* USGS *Woodrow*

FACILITIES: None, though restrooms and a picnic area are at nearby Little Laurel Overlook

WHEELCHAIR ACCESS: None

CONTACT: Marlinton–White Sulphur Ranger District, 304-799-4334

Overview

This hike circles the Tea Creek Backcountry highlands. Start on the Gauley Mountain Trail, then descend the valley of Red Run to Right Fork Tea Creek. Cruise along Right Fork, past beaver dams and meadows, to complete the loop. There are no steep sections, and the trails are well marked and maintained, ideal conditions for novice mountain hikers, including elevation changes less than 500 feet.

Route Details

Begin this trek on the Gauley Mountain Trail, entering the forest to immediately pass a lime-depositing station. Here, lime is fed into the Right Fork of Tea Creek to offset high stream acidity and improve the habitat for native brook trout. Stay right and join an old logging railroad grade. Almost the entire hike traces these grades created to extract timber a century back. Cherry River Boom and Lumber Company and WV Pulp and Paper once owned this land. Timber from here was cut, loaded onto rail cars, then sent either to Cass, West Virginia, for lumber production or Covington, Virginia, to be turned into pulp. Imagine the sounds of trees being felled, loaded, and hauled out over a cleared landscape. Compare that to the now-mature forests exuding sounds of nature, from chirping birds to singing streams to leaves rustling in the breeze.

Wind through a rich forest of spruce, beech, and cherry. Quickly span three small rills on wooden bridges. At 0.4 mile, meet the Right Fork Connector Trail. This is your return route. The handy metal maps that show your position at every trail junction make getting lost a chore. Keep straight on the wide Gauley Mountain Trail. This old grade works gently up the west slope of Gauley Mountain. Open onto a brushy meadow at 1.4 miles. Time will soon overtake this clearing as it has done to other mountain vales. At 2.3 miles, the trail cuts through a gap in a rib ridge of Gauley Mountain. Soon begin a slight downgrade amid spruce and ferns.

Meet the Red Run Trail at 2.7 miles. Turn left on this less-used path, heading west on a very rooty track shaded by red spruce. Come alongside the upper reaches of Red Run at 3.2 miles, sluggishly flowing through this perched valley. You are clearly on an old rail grade. Bridge a tributary at 3.3 miles. Look for the remains of the old rail bridge, collapsed in the streambed. Parts of the path spur off the grade where the former rail line stays wet. Cross another feeder branch of Red Run at 3.6 miles.

Pick your way through a very rocky section of trail as Red Run drops far below in the valley off to your left. The trail steepens a bit, too, then crosses a couple more

Gauley Mountain Loop

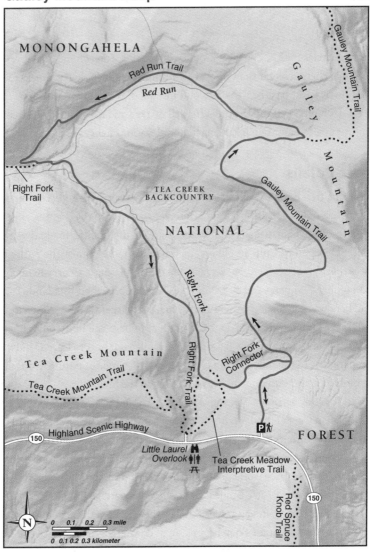

MONONGAHELA

Red Run Trail

Red Run

Gauley Mountain Trail

Right Fork
Trail

TEA CREEK
BACKCOUNTRY

NATIONAL

Gauley Mountain Trail

G a u l e y

M o u n t a i n

Right Fork

Tea Creek Mountain

Tea Creek Mountain Trail

Right Fork Trail

Right Fork
Connector

Highland Scenic Highway

150

Little Laurel
Overlook

Tea Creek Meadow
Interpretive Trail

FOREST

Red Spruce
Knob Trail

150

N

0   0.1   0.2   0.3 mile

0   0.1 0.2 0.3 kilometer

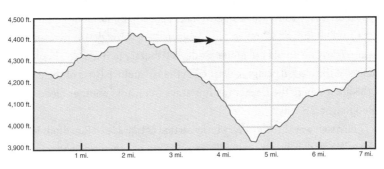

4,500 ft.

4,400 ft.

4,300 ft.

4,200 ft.

4,100 ft.

4,000 ft.

3,900 ft.

1 mi.   2 mi.   3 mi.   4 mi.   5 mi.   6 mi.   7 mi.

feeder branches. The old grade keeps a straight path, then makes a sharp switchback left at 4.5 miles. Descend just a bit more, coming to the Right Fork Trail at 4.6 miles.

Now you reach an especially scenic and interesting hike segment. Stay forward, joining the Right Fork Trail. Rock-hop Red Run, then climb a narrow ridge dividing Red Run from Right Fork. From this ridge you can simultaneously see dark Red Run and translucent Right Fork. At 4.9 miles, rock-hop Right Fork. Pass a massive pool to your left before entering a spruce-bordered field that can be grown head high in late summer. Meadows and beaver dams become a regular feature on Right Fork. Note the skeletal standing trees killed by flooding from beaver dams. Span several small streams on small, wooden bridges. Come to a trail junction at 6.1 miles. For a good view of Gauley Mountain turn right, staying on the Right Fork Trail, and take a short side trip to Tea Creek Meadow.

To finish the loop take the Right Fork Connector Trail, soon passing the Tea Creek Meadow Interpretive Trail. It leads left and right, and is enhanced with interpretive information about the area high country. Continue straight, rising a bit to intersect the Gauley Mountain Trail at 6.8 miles. Turn right on the Gauley Mountain Trail, retracing your steps to reach the Gauley Mountain Trailhead at 7.2 miles, completing your loop.

Nearby Attractions

On this hike you will cross the Tea Creek Meadow Interpretive Trail, an all-access gravel path through high-country meadows. In addition, the auto-accessible Little Laurel Overlook is just a half mile away on Highland Scenic Highway. It offers picturesque panoramas and a picnic table. Additionally, the Tea Creek Mountain Trail starts across the Highland Scenic Highway from the overlook. It offers a single-track natural surface trail that leads 1.7 miles to a view on its way to Tea Creek Campground, yet another attraction that offers shaded, secluded campsites that make a fine base camp for exploring the Tea Creek Backcountry.

Directions

From the Cranberry Mountain Nature Center, 23.0 miles east of Richwood on WV 39/55, head north on Highland Scenic Highway/WV 150 for 17.4 miles to the Gauley Mountain Trailhead, on your left, 0.4 mile after the Little Laurel Overlook. A short gravel road links the highway to the actual parking area.

Alternate directions: From Marlinton, drive north on US 217 for 7.0 miles, then take Highland Scenic Highway/WV 150 west 5.3 miles to the trailhead on your right.

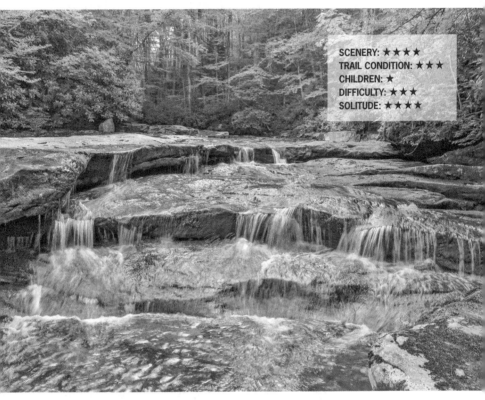

THE FORKS OF TEA CREEK GATHER TO FASHION THIS PICTURESQUE CASCADE.

GPS TRAILHEAD COORDINATES: N38° 20.461' W80° 13.920'

DISTANCE & CONFIGURATION: 7.9-mile loop

HIKING TIME: 4.5 hours

HIGHLIGHTS: Backcountry shelter, Forks of Tea Creek Cascades

ELEVATION: 2,990' at trailhead, 3,800' at high point

ACCESS: No fees or permits required

MAPS: *Tea Creek Area Hiking Trails, Monongahela National Forest;* USGS *Woodrow*

FACILITIES: Campground, restrooms, picnic tables at trailhead, pump well

WHEELCHAIR ACCESS: None

CONTACT: Marlinton–White Sulphur Ranger District, 304-799-4334

Overview

This hike uses the well-marked and maintained trails of Tea Creek Backcountry to travel the valley of Tea Creek to cascades and a trail shelter before looping along the lower slopes of Tea Creek Mountain. Find evidence of logging history in the form of metal relics. Finally, the Tea Creek Mountain Trail takes you back to the trailhead and Tea Creek Campground.

Route Details

This circuit hike exudes beauty with every footfall. The lower Tea Creek valley is especially scenic, with bluffs, big boulders, and shoals. It culminates in Forks of Tea Creek Cascades, a set of tumblers on Right Fork as it flows into Tea Creek, as well as a long slide cascade on Tea Creek itself. Hikers follow old logging grades most of the way, avoiding steep sections, but you will face occasional soggy and rocky trail segments.

Start your loop on the Williams River Trail as it leaves Tea Creek Campground. Follow a straight track over Tea Creek on a 40-foot wooden hiker bridge. Enjoy views of the reddish, rock-strewn mountain brook. Do not take the unsigned user-created trail heading left just beyond the hiker bridge. Instead, continue straight to intersect the signed Tea Creek Mountain Trail at 0.1 mile. Turn left on the Tea Creek Mountain Trail and trace it a mere 80 feet before turning left again on the singletrack Tea Creek Trail. Immediately begin to switchback uphill, rising well above Tea Creek in bouldery hardwoods.

At 0.5 mile, return to Tea Creek and head right, upstream, on an old logging railroad grade that you will trace most of the way. Ahead, frequently step over old meanders created by flooding of ferny bottomlands. Rhododendron-rich islands sporadically stand between you and the creek. Cross a side stream on a wooden bridge at 0.8 mile. The railroad grade is straight and clear. Cut through a fading field at 1.1 miles, then bridge a pair of streams. Wander through an old homesite where rusty tubs and pots are seemingly left for us hikers to find, then cross Lick Creek at 1.5 miles.

At 1.9 miles, travel a stretch of trail where embedded ties from the rail days have been exposed. Just ahead, boulder-strewn Tea Creek on your left and a steep bank on your right pinch in the trail. At 2.2 miles, gaze up to your right at impressive exposed sheer cliffs.

Tea Creek Loop

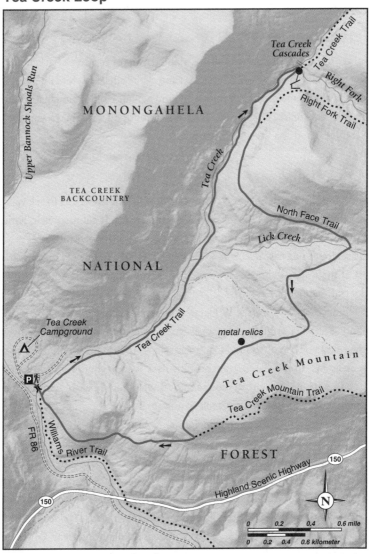

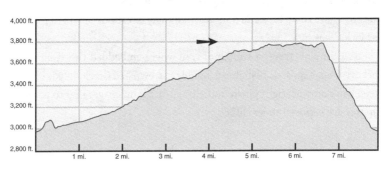

At 2.8 miles, the trail is squeezed in again by the dashing stream to your left and the rising mountainside to your right. Look for a large dark pool in the stream. Just ahead, reach a trail shelter in a small clearing. It is a three-sided Adirondack-style refuge, fronted by a fire ring. A trail leads down to Tea Creek.

The hike continues in front of the shelter. Reach a trail junction at 2.9 miles. Here, the Right Fork Trail leads right and this hike will take it. But first, keep straight and walk a few feet to the scenic confluence of Right Fork Tea Creek and Tea Creek—known as the Forks of Tea Creek. Here, smaller Right Fork drops in a series of short but scintillating falls, then melds into Tea Creek as Tea Creek makes a long slide over an exposed rock slab broken by a wide sunning boulder of massive proportions. Together, the falling waters at this confluence comprise the Forks of Tea Creek Cascades.

After soaking in the scenic waters, join the North Face Trail as it scurries behind the Tea Creek shelter. Begin a mild ascent along an old railroad grade. Pass directly behind the shelter. The wide grade is muddy in spots. At 3.4 miles, reach the Right Fork Trail. Stay straight with the North Face Trail, leaving the sounds of Tea Creek behind. An almost imperceptible uptick takes you to the rock-hop of gurgling Lick Creek at 4.7 miles. Keep winding around the mountainside on the grade. In summer, the brush can be troublesome, so wear long pants. Look for pieces of coal along the former railbed. Aspens grow in great numbers here despite this locale being among the most southern spots in the eastern US where aspens grow. Look for the grayish trunk and the distinctive heart-shaped leaf, then listen for aspen leaves shuttering in the wind.

At 5.5 miles, cross a rocky drainage, then continue curving into the slope of Tea Creek Mountain. Spring branches occasionally cross the trail. At 5.9 miles, come to a concentration of metal relics, perhaps indicating a logging camp or simply some old dump—take note of saw blades, a bed, part of a stove, and some unidentifiable machinery.

The North Face Trail leaves the grade before meeting the Tea Creek Mountain Trail at 6.6 miles. Turn right here, joining a singletrack path that begins a steady descent along the side slope of Tea Creek Mountain. Highland drainages cut across the path. The sounds of the Williams River rise to your ears. Buckeyes increase in number. At 7.8 miles, reach the Tea Creek Trail. From here it is just a short backtrack to Tea Creek Campground and the trailhead.

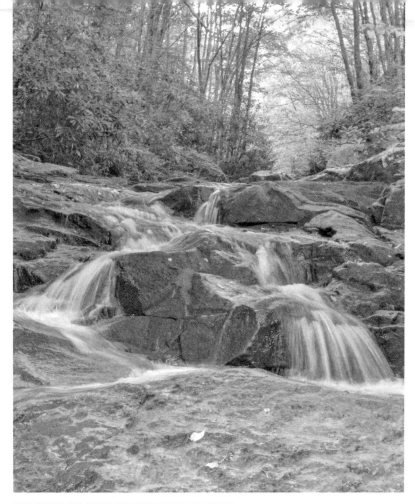

FIND THESE CASCADES ON RIGHT FORK TEA CREEK.

Nearby Attractions

Tea Creek Campground, with its 28 shaded, private, first come, first served sites, makes for a cool and convenient base camp for exploring the trails and waterways of the Tea Creek Backcountry.

Directions

From Marlinton, drive north on US 219 for 7 miles to Highland Scenic Highway/ WV 150. Turn left on Highland Scenic Highway and follow it south 10 miles to Forest Road (FR) 86. Head north a mile on FR 86 to Tea Creek Campground, on your right. The trailhead is on the right just after crossing a bridge over the Williams River at the campground entrance.

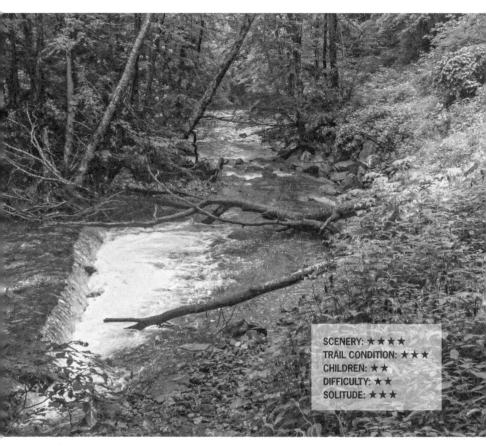

BIG BEECHY RUN COURSES THROUGH JUNGLELIKE FOREST.

SCENERY: ★★★★
TRAIL CONDITION: ★★★
CHILDREN: ★★
DIFFICULTY: ★★
SOLITUDE: ★★★

GPS TRAILHEAD COORDINATES: N38° 33.668', W80° 37.400'

DISTANCE & CONFIGURATION: 5.2-mile out-and-back

HIKING TIME: 3 hours

HIGHLIGHTS: Big Beechy Run Falls, Cranberry Wilderness, Middle Fork Williams River

ELEVATION: 2,410' at trailhead, 2,630' at high point

ACCESS: No fees or permits required

MAPS: *Cranberry Wilderness, Monongahela National Forest;* USGS *Webster Springs SE*

FACILITIES: Primitive campsites, restrooms near trailhead

WHEELCHAIR ACCESS: None

CONTACT: Gauley Ranger District, 304-846-2695

Big Beechy Run Falls

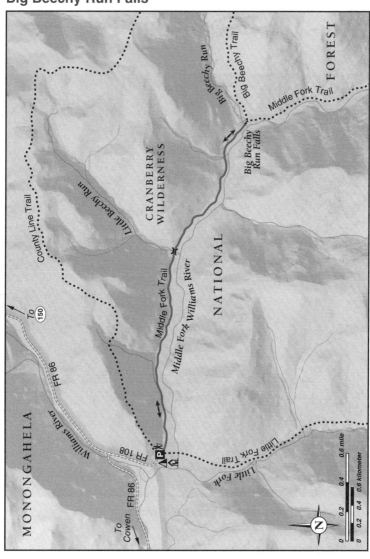

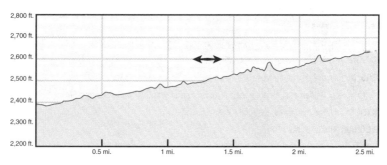

Overview

This hike makes a gentle ascent through the lower Cranberry Wilderness to visit Big Beechy Run Falls, a 10-foot ledge cataract. Though the height of the falls may not seem impressive, the overall scene is worth the walk.

Route Details

This hike traces what once was a forest road before Cranberry Wilderness received its designation in 1983, closing the forest road for good. The forest road was overlaid on an old railroad grade run up Middle Fork Williams River when the valley was logged. Therefore, the route you traverse has transformed from railroad line to auto road to wilderness footpath. The grade is gentle, rising less than 100 feet per mile on its way through the Middle Fork Williams River valley to the mouth of Big Beechy Run, where there is a wide and charming falls with a swimming hole. Big Beechy Run is a tributary of Middle Fork Williams River, and the 10-foot-high falls is the centerpiece of an overall attractive scene. Tall trees, verdant ranks of rhododendron, craggy rock outcrops, and two streams merging and creating light openings in the forest canopy make Big Beechy Run Falls an appealing setting.

Start your hike at the spot known as Three Forks—where the Williams River, Middle Fork Williams River, and Little Fork come together. The U.S. Forest Service has developed designated dispersed campsites near the trailhead. The sites, perfect base camps for exploring the lower Cranberry Wilderness, have a lantern post, picnic table, and a nearby restroom. The first-come, first-served camps are available for a modest fee.

Leave the parking area on the Middle Fork Trail/Forest Trail (FT) #271. The County Line Trail/FT #206 leaves left and ascends. Immediately walk over a stream feeding the Middle Fork. Take a few steps into an overgrown clearing and come to the Little Fork Trail/FT #242, which leaves right to meet the North-South Trail. Continue forward on the Middle Fork Trail, which follows the aforementioned roadbed/railroad grade, now a narrow singletrack path overlain on the grade.

Ahead, pass a trailside kiosk on your left. It includes a map of the Cranberry Wilderness. Parallel a little stream on your left, then cross over a rocky, high-water braid of Middle Fork. A large, wooded flat stretches to your right alongside the Middle Fork. Hike beneath a woodland of tulip trees, yellow birch, and sugar maple. Rhododendron find their place. Hawthorns grow where clearings once stood. Pass near some apple trees at 0.4 mile. County Line Ridge rises sharply to your left.

The walking is easy, though the trailside brush can overwhelm the path in late summer. At 0.8 mile, come near a rising rock bluff to your left. At 0.9 mile, step over a little branch and continue up the grade. At 1.1 miles, a braid of the Middle Fork and a hill to your left pinch in the trail. The main stem of the Middle Fork comes into view on your right at 1.4 miles. Cross a concrete low-water bridge spanning Little Beechy Run at 1.5 miles, then saddle up alongside the Middle Fork. Again, the trail is pinched in by a blasted bluff on your left and Middle Fork on your right. Piled logs and debris in the river indicate the flooding potential of this usually clear mountain stream where trout are often visible in pools below.

BIG BEECHY RUN FALLS LIES IN DEEP, RICH WILDERNESS WOODS.

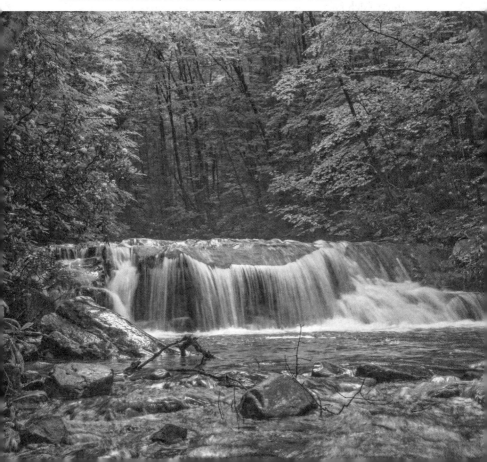

Ahead, pass big boulders on the mountainside and in the stream. The river winds close to and away from the trail. The path is squeezed directly beside the river at 2.1 miles. At 2.3 miles, an old logging road splits left and the railroad grade stays forward.

Enter the valley of Big Beechy Run, reaching the stream itself at 2.6 miles. Backcountry campsites are scattered in the area. Big Beechy Run Falls tumbles just downstream from where the Middle Fork Trail crosses Big Beechy Run. The water from the stream spills over a wide, flat rock slab into a clear plunge pool, ideal for a wilderness dip. This tumbler will be at its finest during late winter, spring, or after a big rain. In summer or autumn, the cascade will show its modest side. Just a few feet below the falls, Big Beechy Run flows into the Middle Fork to form another swimming hole.

Big Beechy Run Falls is the result of a "hanging" valley, created by differing rates of erosion. The primary stream of a valley—Middle Fork in this instance—cuts through the earth faster than tributaries like Big Beechy Run because it carries more water. Eventually, the erosion rate differential between the streams leaves the tributaries "hanging," resulting in a fall at the end of the tributary. Here, at the confluence of Middle Fork and Big Beechy Run, the water of Big Beechy Run has to drop precipitously to meet the Middle Fork, because the waters of Middle Fork have cut deeper into the earth.

Nearby Attractions

The main Williams River offers high-quality trout fishing, including a special catch-and-release area near the trailhead. Also, there are dispersed low-fee campsites along the Williams River and at the Three Fork Trailhead.

Directions

From the Cranberry Mountain Nature Center, 23.0 miles east of Richwood on WV 39/55, head north on Highland Scenic Highway/WV 150 for 13.3 miles to Forest Road (FR) 86. Turn left on FR 86 and follow it 11.5 miles to FR 108, just before the bridge over the Williams River. Turn left on FR 108 and follow it 0.4 mile to dead-end at the Three Forks Area. The Middle Fork Trail starts at the far end of the parking area.

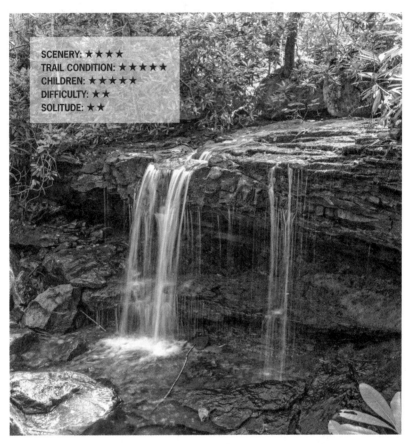

SCENERY: ★★★★
TRAIL CONDITION: ★★★★★
CHILDREN: ★★★★★
DIFFICULTY: ★★
SOLITUDE: ★★

LICK BRANCH FALLS SPILLS IN A CURTAIN FROM AN OVERHANGING LEDGE.

GPS TRAILHEAD COORDINATES: N38° 19.382' W80° 26.308'

DISTANCE & CONFIGURATION: 4.4-mile out-and-back

HIKING TIME: 2.5 hours

HIGHLIGHTS: Cranberry Backcountry, Cranberry River, Lick Branch Falls

ELEVATION: 2,530' at trailhead, 2,620' at high point

ACCESS: No fees or permits required

MAPS: *Cranberry Wilderness, Monongahela National Forest;* USGS *Webster Springs SW*

FACILITIES: Campground, pump well, restrooms at trailhead

WHEELCHAIR ACCESS: Along entire hike

CONTACT: Gauley Ranger District, 304-846-2695

Overview

This hike takes place in the Cranberry Backcountry. Leave a fine national forest campground, then trace a gentle, gated forest road along big and wild Cranberry River. View pools and cascades, then pass a trail shelter before reaching Lick Branch and its waterfall. The walking is easy, so it's great for a family or group hike.

Route Details

The Cranberry Backcountry was established shortly after the Monongahela National Forest came to be. It once covered almost the entire Cranberry River watershed—from Black Mountain in the east to Fork Mountain in the south—a huge swath of remote lands where bears and deer roamed the hollows, trout finned in the streams, and nature reigned supreme. In 1983, the Cranberry Backcountry was divided and much of it became the Cranberry Wilderness. In 2009, the Cranberry Wilderness was expanded, changing designation of additional Cranberry Backcountry to wilderness. This latest change leaves the trail you hike, closed Forest Road (FR) 76, as the boundary of the Cranberry Wilderness. Interestingly, as you hike, terrain to your left is Cranberry Wilderness, while land to your right is Cranberry Backcountry. The entire area is effectively wild and natural. However, while FR 76 is permanently gated and closed to public vehicles, Monongahela National Forest personnel can and do use the road for trail maintenance and the like. Bicyclers like to pedal up the gentle road to fish and explore. However, hikers and backpackers make up the primary trail users.

Leave the parking area and pass around the pole gate up closed FR 76. Remember, only forest personnel can drive this road into the Cranberry Backcountry. Just think of FR 76 as a wide trail extending 16 miles to its northern terminus near the Cranberry Glades. The North-South Trail comes in from your left just beyond the gate, making a long and winding trip from Highland Scenic Highway. The Cranberry River flows strongly to your right as a mix of pools and shoals. Trout fishermen work the river over, especially this close to Cranberry Campground. Walk south in a hardwood forest of beech, birch, and straight-trunked tulip trees, with scattered rhododendron clustering in green groves. The nearly level gravel track makes for easy walking. User-created paths break to fishing holes in the river. Exposed rock opens on the mountainside that rises from the river on your left.

The trail and the river part at 0.4 mile. The Cranberry River has split around an island, as it often does. Come back along the river by 0.6 mile. Note the bluff to your left was blasted to allow passage of a logging rail line and now a forest road.

Lick Branch Falls

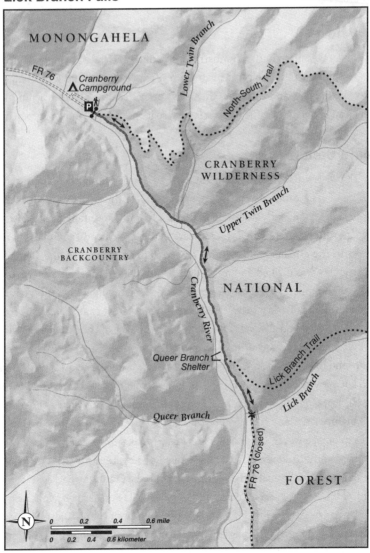

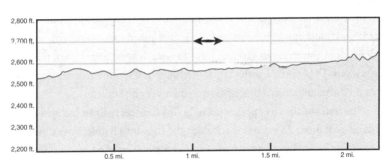

Parts of the track are open to the sun overhead. The track comes along the river and bridges Lower Twin Branch at 0.9 mile and Upper Twin Branch at 1.0 mile.

Ahead, bank up against the ridge rising to your left. This mountain divides the Cranberry River from the Williams River. Continue swinging toward and away from the Cranberry River. At 1.8 miles, come to the Queer Branch trail shelter, located in a flat to your right, facing the Cranberry River. Seven trail shelters are stretched along the Cranberry River. All are accessible from FR 76. These first-come, first-served three-sided wooden huts are open in the front and have a wood floor. Bear food storage cables and a privy are located near each shelter. They are popular during summer, especially on weekends. Campers can find other sites in addition to these shelters along the Cranberry River.

The rerouted Lick Branch Trail leaves left from the shelter area, rising on old logging roads to eventually meet the North-South Trail. Our hike keeps along FR 76, still climbing smoothly. Return to the river's edge before spanning Lick Branch on a bridge at 2.2 miles. Look up the stream to see Lick Branch Falls, a 10-foot curtain-type cascade. A path, the old Lick Branch Trail, allows a closer look at the falls. Here, you can see Lick Branch spill vertically over a ledge. This ledge is undercut, creating a grotto of sorts under the waterfall, where mosses and other moisture-loving plants and amphibians gather. Lick Branch splashes into a rock-littered pool before flowing on and dropping in a second smaller cascade between boulders, then rushing under the forest road and giving its waters up to the Cranberry River. It is an easy backtrack to the trailhead.

Nearby Attractions

Cranberry Campground, located at the trailhead, is an excellent base camp for exploring the Cranberry Backcountry and the lower Cranberry River. The camp offers a mix of shady and sunny campsites spread over a large area and has restrooms and a pump well. All sites are first come, first served.

Directions

From Richwood, drive east on WV 39/55 for 0.5 mile to County Road (CR) 76 (Cranberry Road). Turn left on CR 76 and follow it nearly 3.0 miles to an intersection. Here, FR 76 veers left and is the only gravel road at this intersection. Follow FR 76 for 9.0 miles to Cranberry Campground, on your left just before the road dead-ends. Park at the end of the road, just beyond the campground. The hike starts on the far side of the pole gate.

Falls of Middle Fork

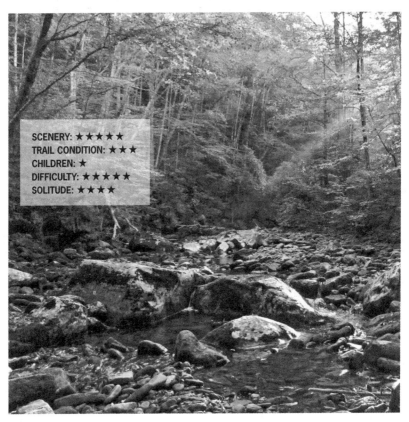

MIDDLE FORK AT LOW WATER

GPS TRAILHEAD COORDINATES: N38° 17.738' W80° 14.915'

DISTANCE & CONFIGURATION: 14.2-mile out-and-back

HIKING TIME: 7 hours

HIGHLIGHTS: Cranberry Wilderness, Hell for Certain Falls, Middle Fork Falls

ELEVATION. 4,240' at trailhead, 2,910' at low point

ACCESS: No fees or permits required

MAPS: *Cranberry Wilderness, Monongahela National Forest;* USGS *Woodrow, Webster Springs SE*

FACILITIES: None

WHEELCHAIR ACCESS: None

CONTACT: Gauley Ranger District, 304-846-2695

Overview

This long out-and-back trek heads into the heart of the Cranberry Wilderness. Trace the Middle Fork Williams River from its highland beginnings to cross multiple tributaries. Mountains rise around you before reaching Middle Fork Falls, a sloped cascade. Continue downriver, then visit the falls on Hell for Certain Branch, a vertical drop that will catch your attention as much as the stream's name does.

Route Details

This hike begins on Highland Scenic Highway at the Big Beechy Trailhead. There you enter the Cranberry Wilderness and cruise through fragrant spruce stands before dipping into the uppermost Williams River valley. From there, a steady but moderate descent leads into a vast hardwood forest, past pools and cascades of the enlarging waterway, crossing tributaries of Middle Fork.

These feeder streams fill Middle Fork Falls, as it makes its river-wide slide into a pool. Downstream, one feeder stream—Hell for Certain Branch—makes its own cataract just before meeting Middle Fork. During the hike, you will experience changing ecotones, from spruce-clad ridgetops to streamside hardwoods.

Pass around boulders blocking old Forest Road (FR) 108, closed way back in in 1983, when the Cranberry Wilderness was established. Trace the former forest road north from the trailhead, on the North Fork Trail. Quickly pass a trail kiosk, then reach a trail intersection at 0.2 mile. Here, the Big Beechy Trail leaves right as a singletrack path, while the North Fork Trail turns south, passing a clearing and then making a nearly level track. Spruce trees crowd the trail, at times forming a tunnel-like canopy.

At 1.3 miles, leave right on the Middle Fork Trail at an intersection. You are still over 4,000 feet but now steadily descending. Make a sharp curve to the right at 1.7 miles, coming alongside the small, upper reaches of Middle Fork. The path can be rocky in places, even though you are following a former fire road. Time and erosion have a way of doing that. The forests, however, have had a century to recover from logging.

At 2.2 miles, the path crosses a rocky braid of Middle Fork. Hardwoods such as yellow birch, beech, and maple become more common. The trail often runs astride the coppery waters flowing over an assemblage of waterworn pebbles, rocks, and boulders. At 3.5 miles, rock-hop North Branch Middle Fork coming in on your right. Continue descending, sometimes through rhododendron coppices.

Falls of Middle Fork

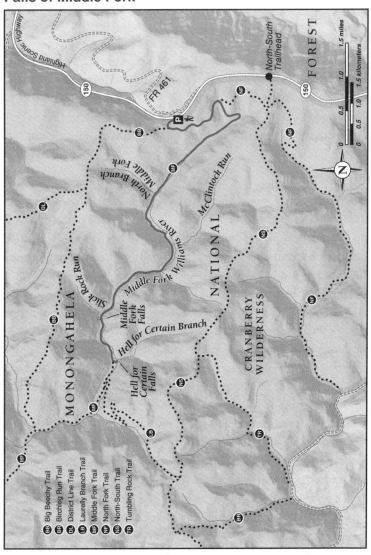

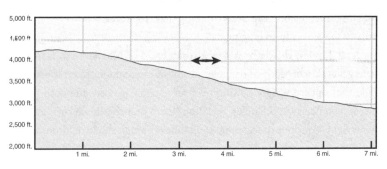

Pools are growing larger in Middle Fork between rapids sliding over rock slabs and dashing between boulders. At 4.6 miles, big McClintock Run enters across the river, giving the valley a wider aspect. You are well above the river. A popular camping area stands on this side of the creek, near some pools and cascades.

At 5.1 miles, you must cross Middle Fork without benefit of a footbridge. This will likely be a wet ford unless the water is very low. Continue downstream, now on the left bank of the river. Come near a huge pool at 5.4 miles, another alluring aquatic scene to be appreciated on the Middle Fork—in addition to the waterfalls.

The spruce are all but gone by this point, but the century-old forest rises in rich splendor of maple, birch, and beech in the bosom of the Cranberry Wilderness. Cross over to the right-hand bank at 5.8 miles. A campsite stands here. At 6.1 miles, the valley widens to your left and Middle Fork is flowing over wide rock slabs. At 6.2 miles, Slick Rock Run splashes over rocks at the trail, where a metal culvert is exposed.

Just beyond this, Middle Fork Falls spills to your left. Here, Middle Fork pours at an angle over a river-wide stone slab, perhaps some 80 feet wide and 10 feet down. This spiller can be quite a sight at high water but is seldom seen then due to the fords required to see it. At lower flows, Middle Fork Falls splits and only flows on along its banks, leaving the center high and dry. The best way to access the cascade is from just downstream of it, where boulders face the falls.

Your Middle Fork adventure continues with easy walking. At 6.9 miles, pass a very conspicuous rectangular boulder in the middle of the trail. Now, be on the lookout for Hell for Certain Falls. At this point, a flat is developing across the river, and is used as a campsite. Hell for Certain Branch flows into the Middle Fork at the lower end of this flat, at 7.1 miles. You must cross the river to see the falls up close, as they are just upstream of a gravel bar where Hell for Certain Branch meets the Middle Fork.

Hell for Certain Falls tumbles about 12 feet over a vertical ledge into a shallow, rocky plunge pool. This perennial stream will be spilling at least a ribbon of water over the ledge. Relax at the nearby campsite after capturing some images of Hell for Certain Falls. The waterfall's name derives from the stream name. I can only imagine some unfortunate woodsman or logger having had a rough experience making their way along the creek. We can now see the falls with comparative ease. Allow plenty of time to make the 7-mile uphill hike to the trailhead.

Nearby Attractions

Tea Creek Campground is just a few miles away from this trailhead and makes a good base camp to explore the Cranberry Wilderness or fish the main Williams River. All sites are first come, first served.

Directions

From the Cranberry Mountain Nature Center, 23.0 miles east of Richwood on WV 39/55, head north on Highland Scenic Highway/WV 150 for 10.2 miles to the Big Beechy Run Trailhead, on your left, across the road from FR 461. The parking area is just a short distance from Highland Scenic Highway/WV 150 on a short gravel track leading to vehicle-blocking boulders. The North Fork Trail begins on the other side of the boulders.

HELL FOR CERTAIN FALLS

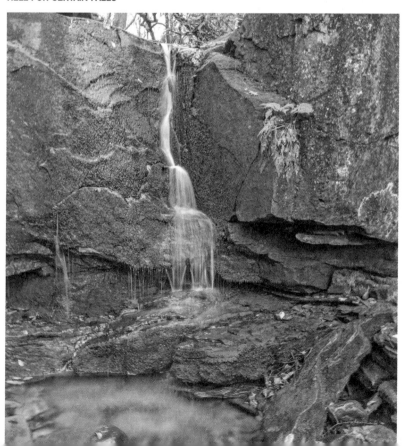

Tumbling Rock Loop

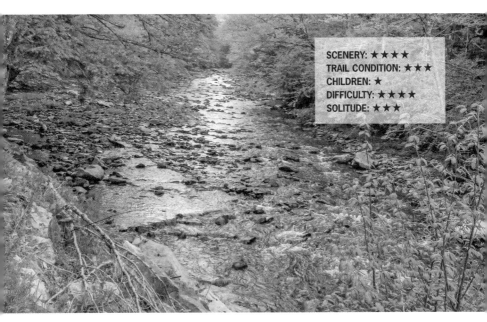

A ROCKY STRETCH OF THE CRANBERRY RIVER.

GPS TRAILHEAD COORDINATES: N38° 16.593' W80° 14.265'

DISTANCE & CONFIGURATION: 16.7-mile balloon

HIKING TIME: 8.5 hours

HIGHLIGHTS: Cranberry Wilderness, backpacking possibilities

ELEVATION: 4,486' at trailhead, 3,075' at low point

ACCESS: No fees or permits required

MAPS: Cranberry Wilderness, Monongahela National Forest; USGS Woodrow, Webster Spring Southeast

FACILITIES: None

WHEELCHAIR ACCESS: None

CONTACT: Marlinton–White Sulphur Ranger District, 304-799-4334

Overview

This classic ridge and stream circuit, an excellent backpack or long day hike, explores the highs and lows of the Cranberry Wilderness. First, traverse the North-South Trail before dropping to the lovely Cranberry River via burbling Tumbling Rock Run. Cruise the riverside, then turn up the North Fork Cranberry River for your return. Campsites and trail shelters enhance overnighting possibilities.

Tumbling Rock Loop

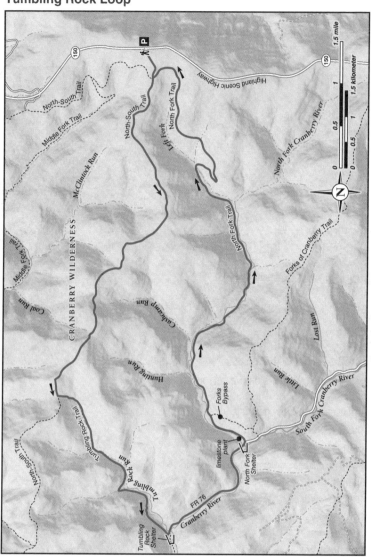

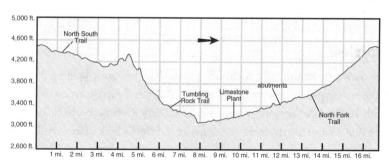

Route Details

The Cranberry Wilderness is a Monongahela National Forest jewel. Since it is a wilderness, trails are lightly maintained. Rock cairns serve as trail markers. This particular hike can be a long day hike or a one- to two-night backpack. Campsites are plentiful throughout the circuit. Leave the scenic highway at 4,500 feet atop Black Mountain and immediately join the east–west running North-South Trail. Veer left, passing a clearing and a trailside kiosk on your left. Keep west through a spruce flat with rocky, rooty footing. Intersect the North Fork Trail at 0.4 mile. The portion of the North Fork Trail to your left will be your return route. Keep straight on the North-South Trail, in an evergreen universe of tall spruce overhead and spongy moss at your feet. Rhododendron and young spruce add more greenery. Expect occasional muddy sections. There will almost surely be some blown down trees to work around. By 2.2 miles, northern hardwoods of yellow birch, cherry, and beech begin to appear on the ridgetop as you gently lose elevation.

The trail veers left at 3.0 miles. Deciduous trees are now common. Descend into a gap at 3.3 miles. Make a couple of more ups and downs, with the final drop to Tumbling Rock Trail traversing rocky woods. Intersect the Tumbling Rock Trail at 5.3 miles. A campsite lies in the gap just ahead. Our loop stays left, descending Tumbling Rock Trail to pick up an old grade. The trail and creekbeds merge in spots, making for messy passage. Notice the railroad ties embedded in the grade at your feet. Feeder branches join here, fashioning a full-fledged water-way. At 6.1 miles, pass through a flat with metal relics, a likely logging camp.

Keep down the valley and cross Tumbling Rock Run at mile 6.3. Leave the grade; you are now following a footpath 100 or more feet above the stream. Swing back to the right and drop to step over a branch of Tumbling Creek at mile 6.9. Climb to a well-graded footpath leading toward Cranberry River. The trail hugs the mountainside and makes a sharp switchback left at an old road, then reaches the Cranberry River at 7.8 miles.

Intersect closed Forest Road (FR) 76. Only official U.S. Forest Service vehicles are allowed passage on this gravel track that marks the Cranberry Wilderness boundary. Turn left up the forest road, quickly bridging Tumbling Rock Run. (Tumbling Rock shelter is to the right a short piece down FR 76.) Parallel the clear and scenic Cranberry River upstream, alternately traversing field and forest, and at times passing directly alongside the Cranberry River.

Reach the North Fork trail shelter on your right at 9.5 miles, a wooden, three-sided refuge with an open front and a nearby privy. Just ahead, span North

Fork Cranberry River, then turn left on the North Fork Trail, soon reaching the Zurbuch Limestone Treatment Plant. Limestone is used to reduce acidity in the Cranberry River, improving trout habitat. Stay to the right of the plant, passing a fine spring on your right.

The trail narrows. Continue up the North Fork Cranberry River, eastbound. Pass the Forks Bypass on your right at 10.2 miles. The North Fork Trail can be overgrown and briery in spots, easy and picturesque in other spots, and mucky in still others. Some sections leave the old grade. Come to old bridge abutments at 11.9 miles. Here, you must rock-hop the North Fork. Briefly pick up the road, then climb left, ultimately heading upstream above washouts before rejoining the grade. Continue up the pretty valley, negotiating tightly grown spruce thickets and passing a couple of campsites.

By 13.3 miles, you are now heading up the small Left Fork Cranberry River valley, rock-hopping the stream at 14.0 miles. Turn back to the southwest, moderately ascending from the vale. The trailbed is open and grassy. At 14.4 miles, dance through a muddy area created by a spring entering from your left. Immediately come to rock cairns signaling a sharp left turn. Quickly rejoin the grade you were just on (the grade made a switchback).

Keep ascending, passing a spring coming in from your right beneath a big boulder at 14.7 miles. Note the USGS benchmark on the boulder. Spruce increase in number as you climb the west flank of Black Mountain, passing spring branches. Intersect the North-South Trail at 16.3 miles. From here, retrace your steps, completing your loop at 16.7 miles.

Nearby Attractions

The Cranberry Wilderness is loaded with other trails, and hikes in this book, including Big Beechy Run Falls.

Directions

From the Cranberry Visitor Center, 23 miles east of Richwood on WV 39/55, head north on Highland Scenic Highway/WV 150 for 8.6 miles to the North-South Trail, on your left.

Alternate directions: From Marlinton, drive north on US 219 for 7.0 miles, then take Highland Scenic Highway/WV 150 south 14.0 miles to the trailhead on your right.

Black Mountain Circuit

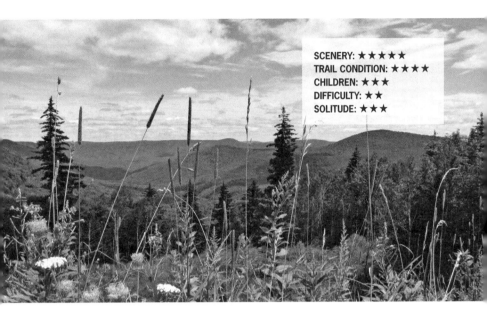

SCENERY: ★ ★ ★ ★
TRAIL CONDITION: ★ ★ ★ ★
CHILDREN: ★ ★ ★
DIFFICULTY: ★ ★
SOLITUDE: ★ ★ ★

LOOKING EAST INTO THE WILLIAMS RIVER VALLEY AND MOUNTAINS BEYOND

GPS TRAILHEAD COORDINATES: N38° 14.808' W80° 14.429'

DISTANCE & CONFIGURATION: 4.8-mile loop

HIKING TIME: 2.5 hours

HIGHLIGHTS: Cranberry Wilderness, high country, interpretive boardwalk, multiple views

ELEVATION: 4,380' at trailhead, 4,520' at high point

ACCESS: No fees or permits required

MAPS: *Cranberry Wilderness, Monongahela National Forest;* USGS *Hillsboro, Woodrow*

FACILITIES: Restroom, small picnic shelter

WHEELCHAIR ACCESS: None

CONTACT: Gauley Ranger District, 304-846-2695

Overview

This high-country hike links two overlooks on Highland Scenic Highway while making a mountaintop walk with highlights aplenty. Hike through woods bordered by fern fields. Grab a view, then emerge onto an interpretive boardwalk, with another panorama. Enter the Cranberry Wilderness, looping back through verdant spruce woods.

Black Mountain Circuit

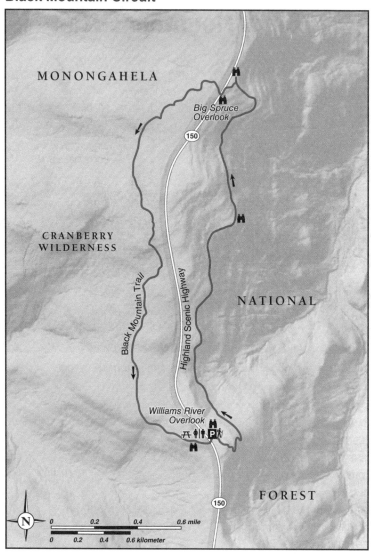

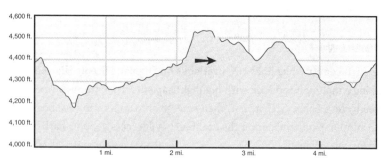

Route Details

Highland Scenic Highway is truly deserving of its name. The road courses through some of the loftiest terrain in the Monongahela National Forest, passing overlooks, trailheads, and campgrounds amid wild, wonderful country. The road starts a few miles north of Marlinton on US 219, then quickly rises to the high country before dropping to cross the Williams River. It then climbs into the heart of the Cranberry area of the forest and heads west along the North Fork Cherry River to end near the town of Richwood after some 43 miles. The roadway is a fine asset that can enhance your Monongahela National Forest experience.

This hike starts at Highland Scenic Highway's Williams River Overlook, standing a shade less than 4,400 feet. To the north, you can see Big Spruce Overlook, the halfway point of this loop, and a host of mountains in the distance. The Williams River valley lies below. Join the Black Mountain Trail behind the overlook restrooms. Climb a bank and actually head south, seemingly the wrong direction, away from Big Spruce Overlook. Traverse mixed woodland dominated by fragrant spruce, and broken with rocks and moss. Listen for the chatter of northern red squirrels as they scold you for entering their domain.

Descend from the ridgetop, slicing between mossy boulders. Drop down the steep east slope of Black Mountain via switchbacks. Don't fret, elevation changes amount to around 300 feet along the course of this hike. The trail is working to get you below the auto overlook's clearing, so you can stay in deep woods. By 0.3 mile, the narrow footpath turns north. Weave among rocks, roots, and trees, which form a lovely forest menagerie for you. The slopes are often clothed in ferns, forming fern banks. Yellow birch, beech, and black cherry represent the deciduous trees. By 0.7 mile, you are going up more than not.

Join an old logging grade at 1.0 mile. The footing is easier, and the vertical variations are lesser. Trees cover much of the level surface, however the trail remains easily passable. Soon, come to a split in the grade. Take the upper grade to your left and continue north. Cross a series of seeps on logs at 1.4 miles. Begin to look for rusty tubs and other implements indicating a former logging camp. The main area of the camp is in an immense fern meadow just past the seep and above the grade. Imagine what it was like to live and work atop this mountain . . . the toil, the danger, the loneliness. The loggers experienced a life far removed from that which we experience today. They would be amazed at the recuperative power of the forest and just how gorgeous it is today.

After leaving the flat, come to a cleared view to your right of Williams River watershed and Big Spruce Knob at 1.5 miles. Highland Scenic Highway and Tea Creek Mountain are visible in the distance. Continue beyond the vista, cruising north, occasionally leaving the grade to work around wet areas. Highland Scenic Highway is well above you yet is never an intrusion. While walking along the grade, look for lumps of coal and rotted crossties.

Suddenly leave the grade to the left at 2.1 miles. Ascend to reach a wooden boardwalk that is part of Big Spruce Overlook at 2.3 miles. Turn right on the boardwalk for another view of Big Spruce Knob and interpretive information about the nature of Black Mountain. Backtrack on the boardwalk through exposed boulders to emerge at Big Spruce Overlook and Highland Scenic Highway at 2.4 miles. Look south toward Williams River Overlook. You just walked from there to here! Stay on the right-hand side of the parking area and cross the highway at the Black Mountain Trail sign.

Enter the 47,000-plus-acre Cranberry Wilderness. This trail courses through its eastern edge. Begin heading southward on a footpath through low trees and open rock spots. Enter deep spruce woods. Make a short, quick descent at 2.9 miles. Roll through forest, then traverse a bouldery, rocky area near the highway at 3.4 miles, dancing between truck-size boulders. Once back in forest, the Black Mountain Trail keeps a steady downward grade for 0.4 mile.

Level off, then climb a hill interspersed with rocks and trees. Look back for views into the Cranberry Wilderness at 4.7 miles. Below you flows the upper reaches of North Fork Cranberry River. Emerge onto the Highland Scenic Highway and the Williams River Overlook at 4.8 miles, completing the circuit.

Nearby Attractions

Forks of Cranberry Trail, a mile south of Williams River Overlook, leads through the Cranberry Wilderness in a young, rock-strewn, fascinating forest, a relic from a long-ago forest fire. Partial views and rock outcrops add to the walk, the first 2.2 miles of which are mostly level.

Directions

From the Cranberry Mountain Nature Center, 23.0 miles east of Richwood on WV 39/55, head north on Highland Scenic Highway/WV 150 for 6.3 miles to the Williams River Overlook, on your right. The Black Mountain Trail starts near the overlook restrooms.

33 **High Rock**

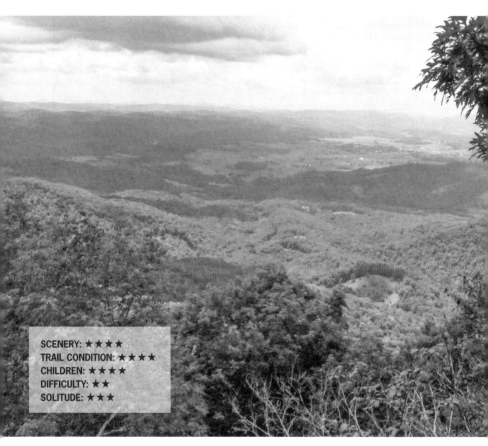

KNOBS AND RIDGES OF WEST VIRGINIA ROLL ON FROM THE HIGH KNOB OVERLOOK.

GPS TRAILHEAD COORDINATES: N38° 12.925' W80° 12.875'

DISTANCE & CONFIGURATION: 3.2-mile out-and-back

HIKING TIME: 2 hours

HIGHLIGHTS: Good views, high country, picnic spot

ELEVATION: 4,300' at trailhead, 4,420' at high point

ACCESS: No fees or permits required

MAPS: *Monongahela National Forest;* USGS *Hillsboro*

FACILITIES: None

WHEELCHAIR ACCESS: None

CONTACT: Gauley Ranger District, 304-846-2695

High Rock

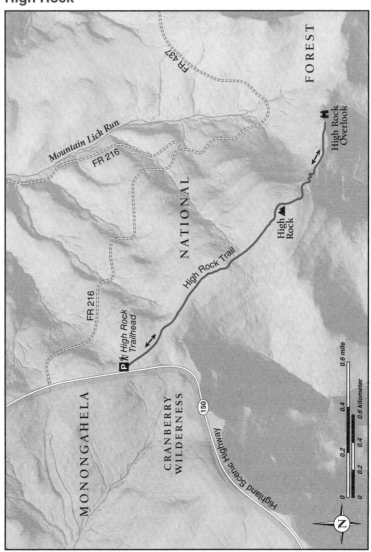

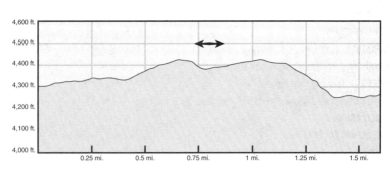

Overview

This relatively easy highland hike leads through an outstanding deciduous forest on a mostly level path to an inspiring overlook. It offers a chance for hikers of all abilities to cruise a lofty ridge leading to a panorama. A shaded, grassy flat at the overlook makes for an agreeable picnic spot.

Route Details

This hike is one of the more popular Cranberry-area treks, as it is doable by all ages and is located near the Cranberry Mountain Nature Center. Leave the Highland Scenic Highway on the well-used High Rock Trail, passing a trailside kiosk, southeast bound. You are tracing a prominent ridge spurring off Cranberry Mountain. Smooth gray trunks of beech trees and taller sugar maples crown the forest. Sugar maple leaves are easy to identify: they have U-shaped notches between their three lobes, as opposed to V-shaped notches between the lobes of red, mountain, and striped maples. Just remember, "sugar maples have a *u* in them." Other big trees along the ridge are northern red oak and buckeye. Interestingly, despite this entire hike being above 4,000 feet, red spruce are noticeably absent from the forest, though you will see a few patches of the evergreen along the way.

The hiking is easy on the singletrack foot trail, crossed with exposed roots. Sawn logs serve as rest benches or places to contemplate nature's beauty. Make a modest uptick at 0.4 mile, then dip to a little gap at 0.7 mile. Pale green ferns swathe the floor of the cathedral-like woodland. In other places, fallen trees have created light gaps. In these light gaps the cycle of growth continues anew, with younger beech, oak, and maple rising for the sky.

At 1.0 mile, top out on the actual knob of High Rock, as noted on official topographic maps, then begin the only significant descent of the hike, just after crossing an old logging road. Even at that, the downgrade only amounts to a little over 200 feet. The trail switchbacks downhill and levels off in a gap at 1.3 miles and continues southeast. At mile 1.6, pass two large oaks in succession just to the right of the path. Soon come to an attractive, grassy clearing shaded by craggy, windswept oaks and ringed on the far side by a wooden fence—this is the High Rock Overlook.

On the far side of the fence an overhanging cliff falls away. As you face outward from the overlook, look for a deep fissure in the outcrop to the left. Layers of rock are exposed on both sides of the fissure. Adventurous explorers follow the cleft in the stone down below the High Rocks. They can't go much farther beyond that, unless they like trail-less wilderness tracking, but it's fun to experience the fissure close up.

The overlook stands at 4,240 feet. The Greenbrier River cuts the valley below—Little Levels valley. You can even see the Greenbrier River glinting in the sun if the light is right. An old railroad grade turned path runs along the river—the Greenbrier River Trail—and it makes for an excellent bicycling adventure. Its southern end starts near Lewisburg, just off Interstate 64. The Greenbrier River Trail follows the old railroad grade up to the town of Cass, an 80-mile journey. Additionally, the Greenbrier is a fun paddling and fishing river.

The villages below the overlook are Mill Point and Hillsboro, which is a little larger and farther to your right. Hillsboro is best known for being the birthplace of noted author Pearl S. Buck. She won the Nobel Prize for literature with *The Good Earth*, her most notable tome, among more than 70 novels. The Allegheny Mountains dividing West Virginia from old Virginia rise in the far east. The nearby mountain is Bald Knob, extending along the same ridge as High Knob.

This is an ideal spot for a picnic, but keep younger hikers under close watch. You may want to look around the outcrop farther than the main view, as other vistas open through the trees to the north of the upper Williams River valley and upper Greenbrier valley amid a sea of ridges that comprise part of West Virginia's montane magnificence.

Nearby Attractions

The Cranberry Mountain Nature Center offers interpretive information, books and maps, a picnic area, and restrooms. It is open Thursday through Monday in season and is located just 3.3 miles south on Highland Scenic Highway/WV 150.

Directions

From the Cranberry Mountain Nature Center, 23 miles east of Richwood on WV 39/55, head north on Highland Scenic Highway/WV 150 for 3.3 miles to the High Rock parking area, on your right. There is room for four or so vehicles.

34 **Cowpasture Loop**

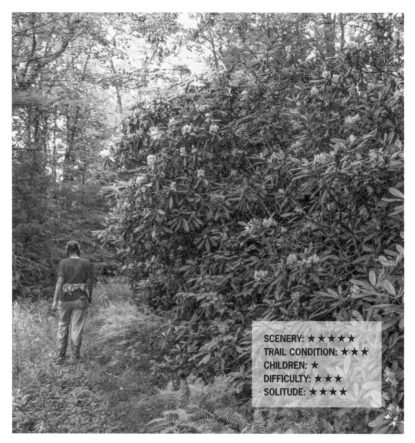

SCENERY: ★★★★★
TRAIL CONDITION: ★★★
CHILDREN: ★
DIFFICULTY: ★★★
SOLITUDE: ★★★★

HIKING THROUGH A RHODODENDRON GARDEN ON THE COWPASTURE LOOP

GPS TRAILHEAD COORDINATES: N38° 11.735' W80° 16.418'

DISTANCE & CONFIGURATION: 7.4-mile loop

HIKING TIME: 4.5 hours

HIGHLIGHTS: Cranberry Glades, varied ecosystems, views galore, World War II prison camp

ELEVATION: 3,400' at trailhead, 3,500' at high point

ACCESS: No fees or permits required

MAPS: *Cranberry Wilderness, Monongahela National Forest*; USGS *Lobelia, Hillsboro*

FACILITIES: None

WHEELCHAIR ACCESS: None

CONTACT: Gauley Ranger District, 304-846-2695

Cowpasture Loop

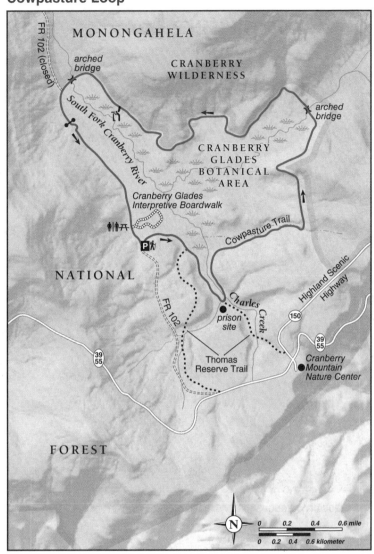

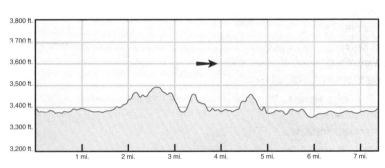

Overview

If you are going to take one hike in the Cranberry Glades area, do this one. The trail encircles unique tundra bogs that lie within this special slice of the Monongahela. In addition to deep spruce woods, hardwood forests, and meadows, it visits a World War II incarceration camp. On top of it all, mountain views are abundant, all while experiencing less than 200 feet in elevation change throughout the circuit!

Route Details

This loop circles the Cranberry Glades Botanical Area. It offers glimpses into a glades ecosystem that is the most southern tundra environment in the country. There are also views of the surrounding mountains as you trace a nearly level course well above 3,000 feet. One open area still has traces of a former federal prison camp where inmates, from moonshiners to those refusing to serve in World War II (conscientious objectors), were housed.

Join the Cowpasture Trail, tracing an old roadbed leading east. Pass a clear area on your left, then enter a northern hardwood forest of black cherry, yellow birch, and maple. The trail is lined with rhododendron. Cross a small branch just before intersecting the Thomas Reserve Trail at 0.5 mile. Keep straight on the level trail and come to a large clearing. Cross a tributary of Charles Creek on a wooden bridge and come to the Mill Point Prison Camp site at 0.9 mile. Ahead, the Thomas Reserve Trail follows old Forest Road (FR) 980 southeast to the Cranberry Mountain Nature Center.

Notice the crumbling blacktop and concrete laid into the clearing. This prison camp had no walls and no cells. The harsh climate and rugged wilderness tamped down thoughts of escape, and violence-prone inmates were not held here. Employees stayed on site, and the prison population, averaging around 300 inmates, worked. The place was nearly self-sustaining, with inmates raising their own food. Mill Point closed in 1959. Just some stone foundations, steps, and a few other relics remain. Explore.

Now turn left, staying on the Cowpasture Trail, and span Charles Creek on a wooden bridge, turning left yet again. The Cowpasture Trail has circled back, now following Charles Creek downstream briefly before resuming an eastern tack. The hiking remains easy, tracing former FR 107 through a rhododendron tunnel and shady woods, with club moss and ferns aplenty. FR 107 was likely preceded by a logging railroad. You are circling the Cranberry Glades to your left. At 2.0 miles, cross another tributary of Charles Creek by culvert, then turn left (north). Bridge another stream at 2.2 miles. Leap over a small ridge, then come to a clearing at 3.0 miles. Kennison Mountain opens above. Watch for a sharp left turn in the clearing at 3.1 miles. Leave the old roadbed, descending through sumacs, hawthorn, and high grass to reach the South Fork Cranberry River at 3.2 miles. Notice the beaver dams on the stream and mountain views into the distance. Climb away from the South Fork Cranberry to rejoin another roadbed, now heading left (southwest).

The trail traverses varied landscapes here, passing through grassy glades, hardwoods, and spruce stands. The habitat variety is amazing. Look for the many hawthorn trees, usually in or near clearings. The short, bushy softwood sports 1-inch thorns on its branches. The trail roughly parallels the boundary of the Cranberry Glades Botanical Area and the Cranberry Wilderness. Both locales are wild and rich in vegetation variety. Cross a wooden bridge at 4.1 miles, continuing moderate ups and downs. Look for more beaver ponds to your left while crossing three more short wooden bridges in succession. Additional mountain panoramas open in meadows.

At 5.3 miles, look left for a side trail leading 0.1 mile to an elevated viewing deck, where you can see more beaver ponds and a host of ridges enfolding the valley. What a view! This is also a good birding spot. Return to the main trail, resuming a path west. Step over more wooden bridges, including a singular arched one over South Fork Cranberry River at 6.0 miles. Leave the waterside willows and enter cool, dark, mossy spruce woods to emerge on gated FR 102. The rich northern hardwood forest shades the road closed to public vehicular traffic, though it is open to bicyclers, equestrians, and hikers.

Turn left on FR 102 and follow it to a gate and the main trailhead for the south end of the Cranberry Backcountry and Cranberry Wilderness, which you reach at 6.3 miles. Continue up gravel FR 102 on a level grade and come to the Cranberry Glades Interpretive Boardwalk, on your left at 7.2 miles. This half-mile side trail explains the unique nature of the Cranberry Glades via informative displays. A small picnic area with restrooms enhances the spot. Beyond the boardwalk continue on FR 102, completing your loop at 7.4 miles.

Nearby Attractions

The Cranberry Glades Interpretive Boardwalk, an all-access loop through the heart of the unique most southern tundra environment in the US, is located just 0.2 mile from the trailhead. Also, the Cranberry Mountain Nature Center is located a short distance from the trailhead.

Directions

From the Cranberry Mountain Nature Center, 23.0 miles east of Richwood on WV 39/55, head west on WV 39/55 for 0.25 mile to paved FR 102. Turn right on FR 102 and follow it 1.3 miles to the Cowpasture Trail, on your right, 0.2 mile before reaching the Cranberry Glades Interpretive Boardwalk parking area.

MOUNTAIN VIEWS AND BEAVER PONDS ENHANCE THE COWPASTURE LOOP.

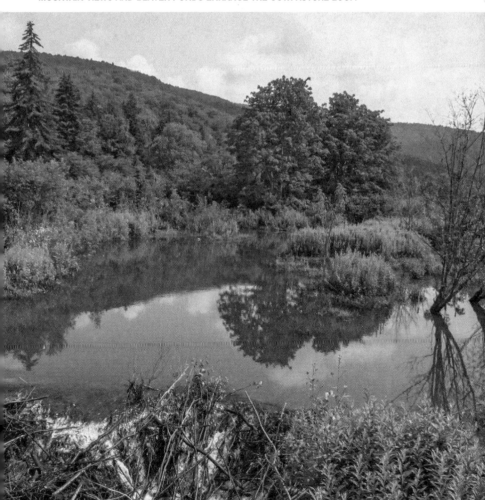

Cranberry Glades
Interpretive Boardwalk

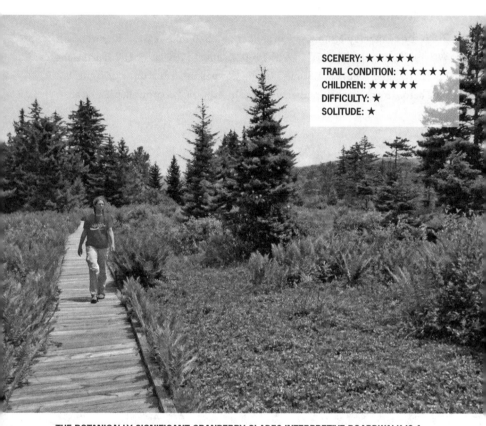

SCENERY: ★ ★ ★ ★ ★
TRAIL CONDITION: ★ ★ ★ ★ ★
CHILDREN: ★ ★ ★ ★ ★
DIFFICULTY: ★
SOLITUDE: ★

THE BOTANICALLY SIGNIFICANT CRANBERRY GLADES INTERPRETIVE BOARDWALK IS A MON MUST-DO WALK.

GPS TRAILHEAD COORDINATES: N38° 11.866 W80° 16.506

DISTANCE & CONFIGURATION: 0.5-mile loop

HIKING TIME: 0.5 hour

HIGHLIGHTS: Botanical interest, tundra-type bogs, views

ELEVATION: 3,380' at trailhead, 3,370' at low point

ACCESS: No fees or permits required

MAPS: *Cranberry Glades Botanical Area, Monongahela National Forest;* USGS *Lobelia*

FACILITIES: Picnic area and restroom at trailhead

WHEELCHAIR ACCESS: Entire loop

CONTACT: Gauley Ranger District, 304-846-2695

Overview

This all-access boardwalk makes a circuit through one of the most botanically important areas of the Monongahela National Forest—the Cranberry Glades. Encircled by high mountains, this sizable highland bog is home to rare plant communities normally seen in Canada. A wooden boardwalk leads through this rare ecosystem. Enjoy viewing the Cranberry Glades plants up close while soaking in mountain views in the distance.

Route Details

The Monongahela National Forest is home to tall mountains, charging rivers, craggy rock outcrops, and an impressive array of flora and fauna. The 750-acre Cranberry Glades Botanical Area, as it is officially known, is perhaps the most treasured complex of flora in the entire national forest. The Cranberry Glades is the largest area of bogs—acidic wetlands found more often in Canada—in the state of West Virginia. The biologically rich wetland is situated in a large bowl surrounded by Kennison Mountain, Cranberry Mountain, and Black Mountain. Here, the headwaters of the Cranberry River form four large named bogs. You can walk by two of them.

Since these are special, protected wetlands, this walk traverses an elevated boardwalk, allowing you to see the plants creating a surface of moss, peat, and precariously growing bog life without damaging the vegetation—or getting your feet wet. Enjoy eight interpretive stops as you wander through a combination of woods, low-slung brush, and low-lying glades. The boardwalk circles Yew Creek, which flows through the heart of the botanical area.

A small picnic area and restroom are located across from the trailhead. Leave the parking area in a mix of rhododendron, hemlock, and spruce. Their roots spread wider than normal in order to survive the shallow, wet soils and high winter winds. After just a few feet, split left and quickly enter Round Glade. Here, the flat peat—created by layers and layers of Sphagnum moss decaying below new moss growth—stretches out and low, availing far views to your north, where Black Mountain looms in the distance with Big Glade and Long Glade lying nearer but well out of reach of this boardwalk. Look for wild cranberry plants growing in Round Glade. Of course, other plants such as ferns, sedges, and grasses mix with the moss and cranberries. It is a designated botanical area after all.

At 0.2 mile, the trail turns right, into an alder thicket. Cross Yew Creek on a boardwalk. Yew Creek is born here in the Cranberry Glades, then feeds its waters to Charlies Creek that in turn flows into the uppermost South Fork

Cranberry Glades Interpretive Boardwalk

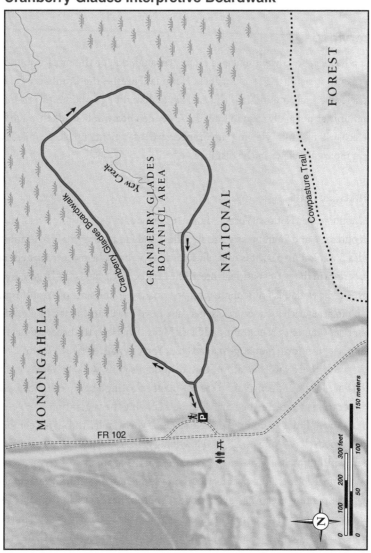

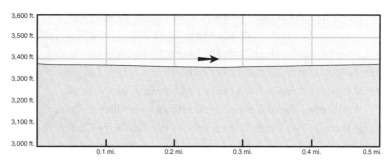

of the Cranberry River. It is from this elevated wetland that the South Fork of the Cranberry River flows, then meets North Fork of the Cranberry River and makes its journey down through the wilderness to meet the mighty Gauley River at Woodbine. And it all starts with trickling Yew Creek and the adjacent bogs that imperceptibly drain the Cranberry Glades.

The all-access trail continues past gigantic ferns. In summertime, the boardwalk can be warm to hot in the sun but cool in the shade of taller trees. Mountain laurel grows where it can find drier ground. Then you enter Flag Glade, another low-slung peat bog. Flag Glade is mostly known for its orchids and sundews. In summer, you may see the blooms of rose Pogonia and grass-pink orchid. The carnivorous sundew and pitcher plants grow here. Both of these insect eaters are popular with photographers when they bloom. June and July are the best times to see and photograph blooming plants in the Cranberry Glades.

After leaving Flag Glade, look for places where small trees are growing atop a fallen log. Here in the Cranberry Glades the challenge for tree growth is not moisture, but too much moisture. The tops of logs form viable tree nursery locales; the rotting wood provides nutrients and a dry place for trees to sprout. Spruce trees pock much of the wetlands.

Also, while on your hike, listen to the rich birdlife attracted to the Cranberry Glades. Cross Yew Creek again before completing the loop portion of the boardwalk. From there it is a short backtrack to the parking area. If you feel like walking more, continue driving down Forest Road (FR) 102 for 1 mile to a turnaround and parking area. Here, you can follow the gated road downstream through spruce and hardwoods along the upper South Fork. Another option is to hike part of the Cowpasture Trail, accessible just south of the Cranberry Glades parking area.

Nearby Attractions

Cranberry Mountain Nature Center, just a short drive from this trailhead, offers additional interpretive information about the Cranberry Glades. Additionally, the Falls of Hills Creek hike, also detailed in this guide on pages 178–181, is just a few miles west down WV 39/55. Campers can overnight at Summit Lake, located off WV 39/55 west of the Cranberry Glades.

Directions

From the Cranberry Mountain Nature Center, 23.0 miles east of Richwood on WV 39/55, head west on WV 39/55 for 0.25 mile to paved FR 102. Turn right on FR 102 and follow it 1.5 miles to the Cranberry Glades parking area, on your right.

Falls of Hills Creek

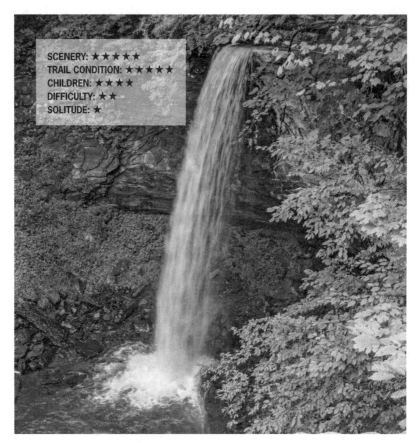

LOWER FALLS CHARGES OVER AN UNDERCUT ROCK HOUSE.

GPS TRAILHEAD COORDINATES: N38° 10.700' W80° 20.328'

DISTANCE & CONFIGURATION: 1.6-mile out-and-back

HIKING TIME: 1 hour

HIGHLIGHTS: Impressive trail construction, three exciting waterfalls

ELEVATION: 3,450' at trailhead, 3,260' at low point

ACCESS: No fees or permits required

MAPS: *Falls of Hills Creek, Monongahela National Forest;* USGS *Lobelia*

FACILITIES: Vault restrooms

WHEELCHAIR ACCESS: First 0.3 mile of trail

CONTACT: Gauley Ranger District, 304-846-2695

Overview

This hike leads you to three impressive cataracts within the Falls of Hills Creek Scenic Area. Start on a paved all-access path and cruise past big trees to the 25-foot Upper Falls. Beyond the first waterfall trace is an impressive and costly trail using wood and metal to allow access to Middle and Lower Falls in a deep, wild gorge. Lower Falls is West Virginia's second-highest cataract at 63 feet.

Route Details

Many waterfall lovers have no idea what an elaborate trail they are going to follow to make the triple cataract crown of Hills Creek. Leave the parking area on the all-access asphalt Falls of Hills Creek Trail. Enter rich woodland of spruce, yellow birch, maple, and beech, all components of the northern hardwood forest. Striped maples are a common understory tree here and have leaves resembling a goosefoot and vertically striped bark. Striped maples rarely grow taller than 25 feet. At 0.1 mile, the natural-surface Fork Mountain Trail veers right as the Falls of Hills Creek Trail makes a very sharp left turn. A shortcut heads right, skipping Upper Falls. Most hikers return to the trailhead using this shortcut, after they have visited the three falls.

Rosebay rhododendron forms vast thickets. Its pinkish-white blooms color the scenic area in July. Hemlock, preserved along this trail, adds greenery. Continue winding toward Hills Creek on a wheelchair-compliant grade. Ahead, the other end of the Fork Mountain Trail leaves left to cross Hills Creek. At 0.3 mile, come to the Upper Falls Overlook. Upper Falls dives 25 feet off a ledge enveloped by hemlock trees. Here, as it is throughout the gorge, Hills Creek has flowed over hard sandstone, eventually cutting through to the softer shale below. When the shale eroded, it couldn't support the harder sandstone and the sandstone collapsed, deepening the gorge over time. This overlook is well above Upper Falls, making it difficult to see the face of the fall.

The wheelchair-accessible segment of this trail ends at Upper Falls. Continue on a gravel and wood path, passing a shortcut back to the parking lot on your right. Soon reach a wooden boardwalk built into the steep slope of the mountainside, which in summer can be overgrown with stinging nettle. Be careful after rains or when frozen, this boardwalk can be slick! Use the handrails. The boardwalk drops into the gorge using many steps.

Leave the boardwalk at 0.5 mile and resume a gravel footpath. Open onto a flat where yellow birch rise above groves of rhododendron. Hills Creek

Falls of Hills Creek

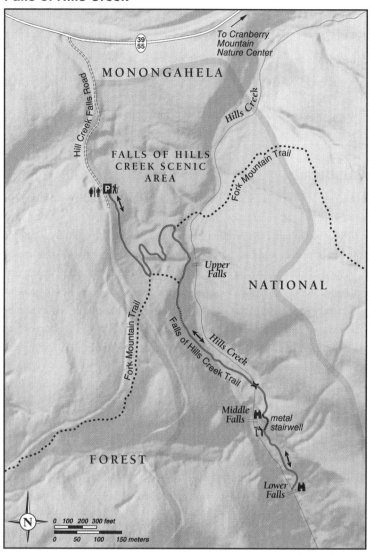

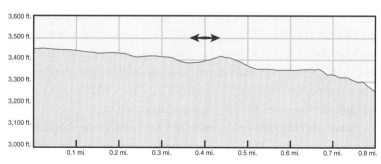

continues its downgrade, alternating in pools and shoals. Span an attractive arched footbridge over Hills Creek, leaving the bridge on a stone slab. Soon come to a viewing platform of wide Middle Falls on your right. This platform looks down on the watery 45-foot cataract as it spills over an irregular and jagged ledge. Leave this platform, then reach a wide deck. Just beyond the deck, descend a metal stairwell astride a rock bluff. Look at the layers of the bluff while descending, as well as the construction of the deck and metal stairs. This metal contraption leads to a spur and another platform, offering a bottom-up view of the Middle Falls. Here, you face the falls as it lurches wide over the ledge, briefly gathers in a pool, then powers forward down a rock jumble, ultimately coursing past the platform and on through the gorge.

Continue downstream on Hills Creek via another wooden boardwalk. The walls of the rock bluff rise on both sides of the creek. Short-lived waterfalls will pour over sides of the bluff following thunderstorms. View Lower Falls on your right as it plunges from a stone lip into the void below—at least that's the view from this vantage. A more complete look lies ahead. Descend another set of wooden steps to view Lower Falls. This cataract is as narrow as Middle Falls is wide. It nosedives 63 feet down from an overhanging bluff into a semicircular stone amphitheater, bubbling into a white froth and a circular pool. No trails lead to the bottom of the falls. The land falls steep and brushy from the deck.

Lower Falls is West Virginia's second-highest fall. The return trip requires a little more effort than it took to get there. Take the time to contemplate and appreciate the elaborate trail construction that makes seeing these falls possible.

Nearby Attractions

Cranberry Mountain Nature Center is just 5 miles east of the Falls of Hills Creek Scenic Area. It offers interpretive information, maps, and more in season. Hiking-wise, a 0.5-mile boardwalk makes a level and view-filled circuit through the Cranberry Glades Botanical Area.

Directions

From the Cranberry Mountain Nature Center east of Richwood and west of Marlinton, drive 5.2 miles west on WV 39/55 to the Falls of Hills Creek Scenic Area on your left.

37 Summit Lake Loop

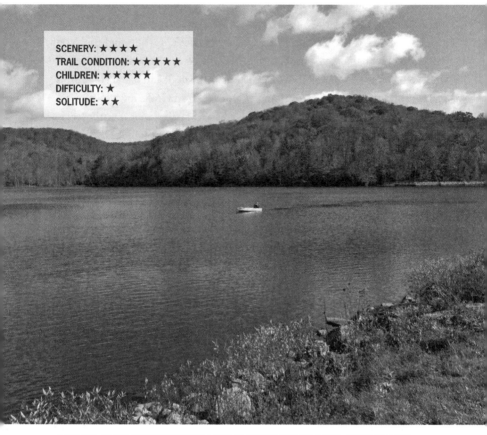

SCENERY: ★ ★ ★ ★
TRAIL CONDITION: ★ ★ ★ ★ ★
CHILDREN: ★ ★ ★ ★ ★
DIFFICULTY: ★
SOLITUDE: ★ ★

A BOATER TOOLS AROUND SUMMIT LAKE AS SEEN FROM THE TRAIL AS IT CROSSES THE LAKE'S DAM.

GPS TRAILHEAD COORDINATES: N38° 14.987' W80° 26.071'

DISTANCE & CONFIGURATION: 1.7-mile loop

HIKING TIME: 1 hour

HIGHLIGHTS: Boardwalks, lake views, multiple recreation opportunities

ELEVATION: 3,405' at trailhead, 3,430' at high point

ACCESS: No fees or permits required

MAPS: *Cranberry Wilderness, Monongahela National Forest;* USGS *Fork Mountain, Webster Springs SW*

FACILITIES: Boat ramp, campground, picnic area, restroom

WHEELCHAIR ACCESS: On boardwalk/fishing pier

CONTACT: Gauley Ranger District, 304-846-2695

Overview

This walk, suitable for the entire family, takes you around the highland impoundment and recreation area near Richwood. Walk along a wooden boardwalk over the lake, then join a footpath circling 43-acre Summit Lake. Cross Coats Run and its tributaries before paralleling the shoreline, availing aquatic and montane views. Complement your walk with other activities such as picnicking, paddling, fishing, and camping.

Route Details

The name Summit Lake seems appropriate after the elevation-gaining drive up from Richwood. There are no natural lakes in the Monongahela National Forest, but Summit Lake enhances the expected mountain finery of hills, hollows, forests, and streams. Here in the Yew Mountains, where Coats Run—a tributary of North Fork Cherry River—has been dammed, a 43-acre lake now reflects the surrounding hills and adds another physical feature to the Monongahela National Forest.

Summit Lake Recreation Area has not only hiking trails but also a fine 33-unit campground. And where you have water you often have fishing. The West Virginia Department of Natural Resources stocks the highland tarn, attracting anglers who bank fish and endeavor, in boats and canoes and kayaks, to catch fish. Beneath the surface swim all manner of finned fare: brook trout, brown trout, rainbow trout, largemouth bass, and crappie. Since no gas motors are allowed on Summit Lake, this leaves a quiet experience while on—or near—the water.

For on this hike you will be near the lake nearly every step of the way. Your first steps should be on the wooden boardwalk/fishing pier that runs parallel to the graveled Summit Lake Trail. You may have to elbow your way past some anglers, but the views and closeness to the water are worth it. Soon join the official Summit Lake Trail. The gravel track has been running parallel to the boardwalk.

Travel along the shoreline under beech, maple, and Fraser magnolia, with scattered pockets of rhododendron. Good views into the lake frequently open. User-created spur trails allow direct water access. Pass an observation bench, then turn into one of two coves on upper Summit Lake. Bisect rhododendron thickets, then cross Coats Run on a wooden hiker bridge at 0.5 mile. This stream feeds cold, clear mountain water from a steep ridge dividing Coats Run and the Cherry River watershed from the Cranberry River watershed.

Summit Lake Loop

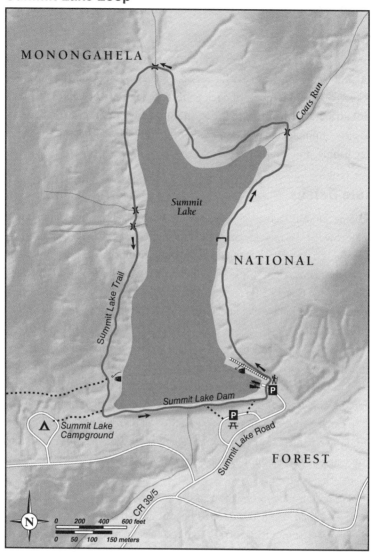

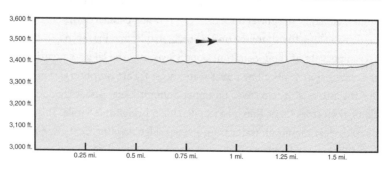

Circle around the cove and return to the shore, where a grassy point allows a southward vantage of Summit Lake Dam making a horizontal line in the distance. Summit Lake Trail turns into the second cove and bridges an unnamed feeder branch flowing from the knob of Hanging Rock at 0.8 mile. Elevation changes are nearly nonexistent on the walk as you turn back south on the west side of Summit Lake. Beech trees grow dense here. Oaks rise tall and club moss is a prevalent ground plant.

At 1.0 mile, pass a pair of bridges spanning seasonal streams. Short boardwalks cover other potentially wet areas. By 1.2 miles, the hillside has risen to your right. Note artificial land piers extending into Summit Lake. These provide fishing access. At 1.3 miles, reach the first of two spur trails leading right to the recreation area campground.

Summit Lake Campground, open April through November with first come, first served campsites, has two loops. The loop closest to the Summit Lake Trail is smaller. It has nine campsites, tiered and leveled into a mountainside. Seven of the nine campsites are on the inside of the loop. Each campsite pull-in is paved. Each graveled area houses a picnic table, fire grate, and lantern post. A set of vault toilets and a water spigot lie on the outside of the loop.

The second loop is farther from the lake and is also linked to Summit Lake by its own trail. Twenty-four well-spaced campsites make this a much bigger and more active part of the campground. The campsites, mostly on the outside of the loop with nice views into the surrounding woods, are also cut into the mountainside and leveled. Some of the campsites are pull-through.

The aforementioned campground access trails also link campers to a shoreline fishing dock. At 1.4 miles, the Summit Lake Trail turns left (east) and begins crossing the arrow-straight, grass-covered dam holding back the waters of Summit Lake. Watery views really open up here as you make the final leg to the trailhead and boat ramp. Pass a couple of spur trails dropping from the dam to the picnic area. Soon you are across the dam and back to the boat ramp and parking area, completing the circuit hike.

Nearby Attractions

The Cranberry Glades are located east of Summit Lake on WV 39/55 and have a fine boardwalk through a special wetland with extensive views of the adjacent mountains. Also, the Cranberry Mountain Nature Center is just a little farther on WV 39/55 than the Cranberry Glades. The visitor center offers interpretive information about the Monongahela and greater Cranberry area. Finally, the Highland Scenic Highway extends north from the Cranberry Mountain Nature Center and has multiple auto-accessible overlooks and trailheads for other hikes.

Directions

From Richwood, drive east on WV 39/55 for 7.2 miles to County Road (CR) 39/5 (Summit Lake Road) just after passing North Bend Picnic Area. Turn left on CR 39/5 and climb 2.1 miles to Summit Lake. Follow the main road, then split right toward the boat launch. Park in the boat launch parking area. The signed Summit Lake Trail starts near the boat ramp.

A VIEW OF THE FISHING PIER ON SUMMIT LAKE

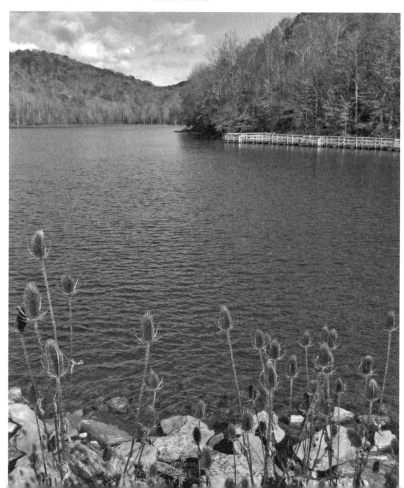

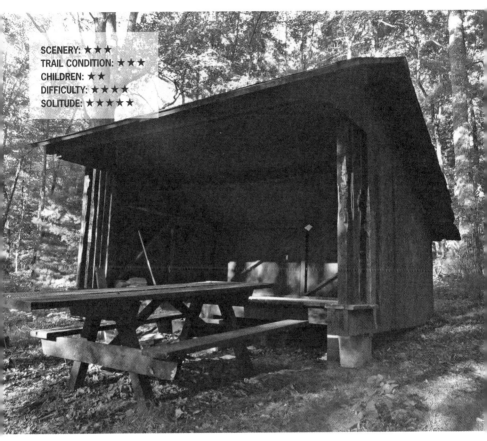 38 Laurel Creek Circuit

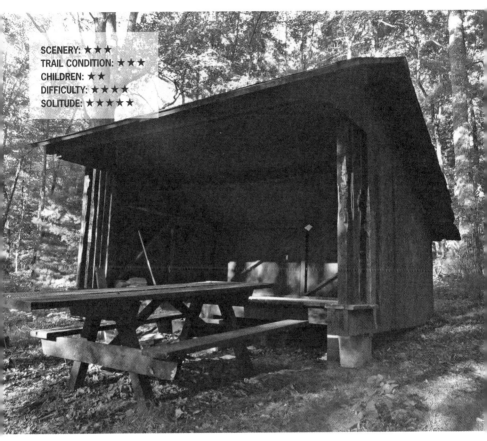

SCENERY: ★★★
TRAIL CONDITION: ★★★
CHILDREN: ★★
DIFFICULTY: ★★★★
SOLITUDE: ★★★★★

THE TRAIL SHELTER ON LOCKRIDGE MOUNTAIN IS A WELCOME SIGHT.

GPS TRAILHEAD COORDINATES: N38° 07.661' W79° 57.413'

DISTANCE & CONFIGURATION: 8.5-mile loop

HIKING TIME: 4.5 hours

HIGHLIGHTS: Solitude, streamside environment, trail shelter

ELEVATION: 2,440' at trailhead, 3,000' at high point

ACCESS: No fees or permits required

MAPS: *Monongahela National Forest;* USGS *Minnehaha Springs*

FACILITIES: Campground nearby, picnic area at trailhead, restrooms

WHEELCHAIR ACCESS: None

CONTACT: Marlinton–White Sulphur Ranger District, 304-799-4334

Laurel Creek Circuit

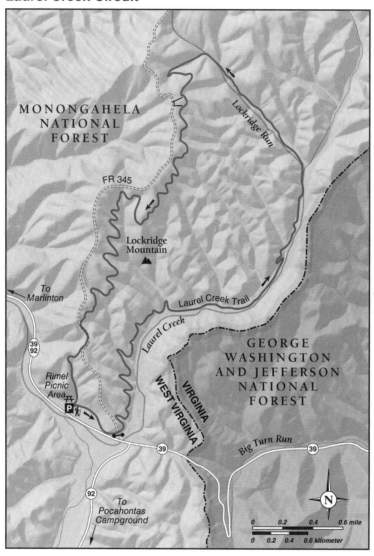

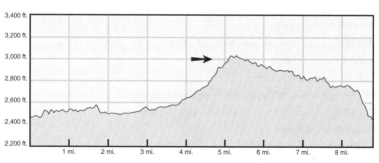

Overview

This seemingly forgotten and certainly underutilized loop hike is worth your time, especially for solitude seekers. Leave Rimel Picnic Area near Minnehaha Springs, then hike astride the West Virginia–Virginia border along scenic Laurel Creek before climbing Lockridge Mountain via Lockridge Run. Complete the loop by winding in and out of hollows on Lockridge Run. The hike is easier than its 8.5 miles may seem—the trail is well graded and has only a 600-foot elevation difference between its low and high points. However, allow plenty of time to cover the entire loop.

Route Details

Join the Laurel Creek Trail at the upper end of the Rimel Picnic Area, next to an informational kiosk with trail information, walk just a few feet, and turn right, beginning your circuit. Immediately cross a wooden boardwalk to enter a regenerating forest. The track heads east, roughly paralleling WV 39/92, while crossing closed Forest Road (FR) 345. The singletrack path then turns north into the Laurel Creek watershed, beginning a pattern of winding in and out of hollows with Lockridge Mountain rising to your left and Laurel Creek below to your right.

The streambeds at the base of the hollows are intermittent, yet wooden bridges have been erected over the streams for times of flow. The first such bridge is encountered at 0.8 mile. Cross others at 1.0, 1.3, 1.8, and 1.9 miles. The flat of Laurel Creek and small clearings are visible below while working around rib ridges between the hollows.

Elevation changes are negligible as the trail meanders farther into Laurel Creek valley. At 2.0 miles, the path reaches the valley floor and an old railroad grade, and is more level than before and much straighter. Tall pines tower over rhododendron, ferns, and maples. Laurel Creek flows nearby to your right, and you gain glimpses of the clear, stony trout stream. The West Virginia–Virginia border is formed by the low ridge across Laurel Creek. This low ridge divides Laurel Creek drainage from Little Back Creek in the Old Dominion.

The railroad grade crosses intermittent streams emanating from side hollows. Even when flowing, these streams can be easily crossed. Trailside wildlife clearings offer open contrast in the wooded valley. Continue up the large flat. The wide trail allows you to appreciate your surroundings and not have to stare down, negotiating every footfall. Ahead, Laurel Creek braids, forming islands in the stream. Blue blazes lead across the braids. Young beech trees border the path on these islands. In places, the old railroad grade has been partially washed out.

At 2.9 miles, the Laurel Creek Trail leaves the grade, using a reroute working around a mucky bottom. At 3.4 miles, leave Laurel Creek and turn left, up Lockridge Run, while the grade keeps forward along Laurel Creek. This side stream mimics Laurel Creek in many ways, yet has a steeper gradient, as side streams usually do. Lockridge Run has its own feeder branches that push across the trail in places. Step over Lockridge Run six times while the valley narrows.

After the sixth crossing, the loop trail steepens and splits left up a normally dry tributary of Lockridge Run. Switchbacks lead to the crest of Lockridge Mountain, cloaked in oak woods. The path takes a southern direction along the east side of the mountain and reaches a spur trail at 5.3 miles. Here, the spur trail leads uphill a short piece to a trail shelter. The three-sided Adirondack-style wooden refuge has a picnic table and makes a good stopping point, especially since you are at the hike's high point. Water can be had from the spring-fed wildlife pond located below the Laurel Creek Trail near the spur trail junction.

Beyond the shelter, the trail resumes its pattern, keeping on the east side of Lockridge Mountain, winding around the upper ends of hollows, with little vertical variation. At 6.4 miles, the path conspicuously curves back to the north and then resumes its southern ways and the hollow-rib ridge pattern, imperceptibly working downhill. Winter views open of the Virginia mountains to the east. At 8.2 miles, the trail crosses closed FR 345. Look for a small pond to your right just after crossing the forest road. The path parallels the forest road before diving into a slender stream defile, emerging at Rimel Picnic Area to complete the loop at 8.5 miles.

Nearby Attractions

Pocahontas Campground, located about a mile south of Rimel Picnic Area on WV 92, is a great base camp for hiking the Laurel Creek Trail. Pocahontas is an extremely pretty campground set in a forest of giant white pine beside a valley stream; it is little used, inexpensive, and has quiet, yet well-maintained, mountain biking and additional hiking trails leaving directly from the first come, first served campground open from mid-March through November.

Directions

From Marlinton, drive east on WV 39/92 for 12.6 miles to reach the Rimel Picnic Area, on your left. The picnic area is before the intersection where WV 92 splits off to the right. The Laurel Creek Trail leaves directly from the upper end of the parking area.

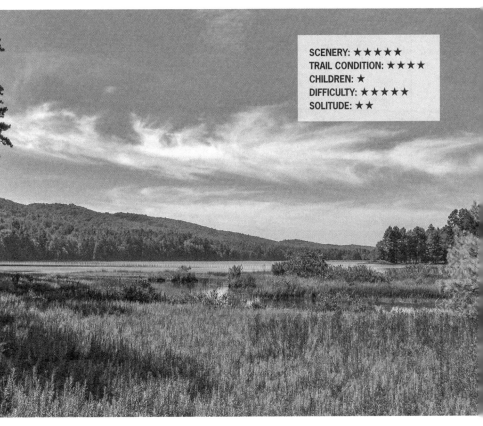

LOOKING SOUTH AT LAKE SHERWOOD

GPS TRAILHEAD COORDINATES: N38° 0.393' W80° 0.875'

DISTANCE & CONFIGURATION: 10.6-mile loop

HIKING TIME: 5.5 hours

HIGHLIGHTS: Diverse environments, lake views, mountain views

ELEVATION: 2,670' at trailhead, 3,200' at high point

ACCESS: Entrance fee required during warm season

MAPS: *Lake Sherwood Area Hiking Trails, Monongahela National Forest; USGS Lake Sherwood, Mountain Grove, Falling Spring, Rucker Gap*

FACILITIES: Campground nearby, picnic area at trailhead, restrooms

WHEELCHAIR ACCESS: None

CONTACT: Marlinton–White Sulphur Springs District, 304-536-2144

Lake Sherwood Loop

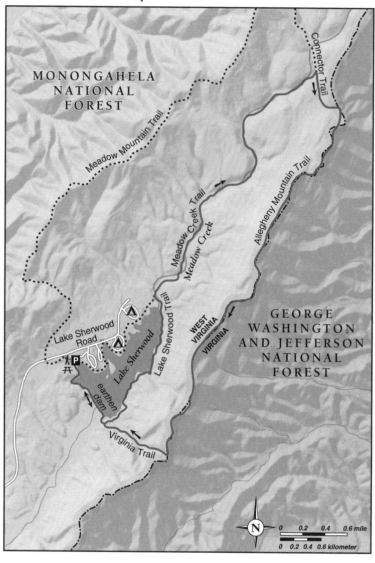

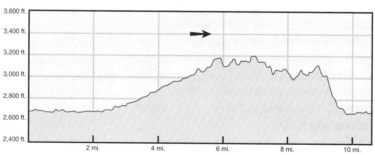

Overview

This stellar loop hike traverses three distinct environments. Start your trek on the shores of Lake Sherwood, West Virginia's prettiest lake. Then make a streamside walk along Meadow Creek. Climb up to the high ridge that forms the boundary between West Virginia and Virginia. Travel south along the state line and enjoy views into both states before returning to Lake Sherwood.

Route Details

Do not let the mileage scare you from doing this hike. Not only is the hike a winner, but the entire Lake Sherwood Recreation Area is a fine place to spend your time. There are very few steep sections on the state line ridge, and the ascent from Lake Sherwood to the state line is very gradual. The main challenge is the mileage. Take your time and make a day of it. Be aware there is no more water available after you leave Meadow Creek.

You are nearly certain to have company along Lake Sherwood, but after that the loop will probably be yours. Leave the parking area at the picnic area turnaround loop on the Lake Sherwood Trail and immediately cross a little wooden footbridge. Quickly reach a trail junction. Turn right and begin tracing the wooded shore of Lake Sherwood, on your left, as you gain good lake views. Swing around a cove and come to the lake dam at 0.5 mile. Keep straight and cross the earthen dike while soaking in fantastic vistas of the mountain impoundment and Meadow Creek Mountain on your left.

Cross over the spillway bridge and reach the Virginia Trail, your return route, at 0.8 mile. Stay left on the Lake Sherwood Trail, beginning the loop portion of the hike. The white pine–dominated woodland presents nearly continuous views into the mountain-framed lake as you undulate over small hills dividing mostly dry streambeds. Relaxation and repose benches beckon alongside the trail. Spyglasses offer views of the swim beach and campground across the impoundment.

Meet the Meadow Creek Trail at 2.2 miles, just before the footbridge over Meadow Creek. If you desire a shorter trek, just follow the Lake Sherwood Trail left to complete a circuit around the lake, passing by the camping area along the way. Our loop turns right on the Meadow Creek Trail. Begin a moderate ascent alongside the alluring evergreen-shrouded stream. Pinewoods tower overhead. Make the first of many creek crossings in 0.3 mile. These can all be easily rock-hopped in times of normal flow, especially with the placed stepping-stones.

Make four more fords in the next mile. Note both Catawba and rosebay rhododendron grow here.

The creek crossings continue as Meadow Creek becomes ever smaller. Vegetation crowds the path, making the walk seem a jungle trek at times. Emerge onto an old woods road at 5.1 miles. This is the Connector Trail. Turn right on the Connector Trail and leave the rhododendron behind. An oak-hickory forest rises above an understory rife with mountain laurel.

Soon reach a game clearing. Head directly across the grassy field, then look for the blue blazes at the clearing's end, slightly to your left. Come to the Allegheny Mountain Trail and the state line at 5.6 miles. Turn right on the Allegheny Mountain Trail, heading upward and south along an old fire road, originally built by the Civilian Conservation Corps in the 1930s. It has all but devolved to a hiking trail these days, however.

Begin rolling up and over small knobs and down to gaps among the hickories and oaks. Note the countless blueberry bushes along the trail, which will be ripe with fruit in late July. Also, look overhead at the many large acorn-bearing oaks that, along with the blueberries, provide abundant food for wildlife. Measure how much steeper the drop-off is on the Virginia side of the ridge, as opposed to the gentle slopes here in the Mountain State.

At 6.3 miles, the Allegheny Mountain Trail dives off the ridge to your right. This is the only very steep section of the loop and it ends quickly. Swing around the right side of a rock house. Just past this rock house, you can climb this very outcrop to your left and garner some rewarding panoramas of Virginia's Blue Ridge.

Keep southward, riding the knife-edge rock uplift. The treadway is tough, but the views into both states demand a slow pace. Eventually, the ridge widens out and the trail becomes more foot friendly. At 7.7 miles, in a gap, look for Lake Moomaw to your left. This is a recreation area in Virginia's George Washington and Jefferson National Forest, much like Lake Sherwood.

Ahead are still more views of Lake Moomaw. At 8.5 miles, the trail widens as an old road comes in from your left. Stay straight and begin the most continuous climb of the hike. Top out on a knob, and descend to the Virginia Trail at 9.2 miles.

At the intersection, an old woods road keeps straight to a partial view. Our hike turns right on the Virginia Trail and drops steeply. The descent moderates when it picks up an old wagon road and parallels a streambed to your right. Turn away from the stream. Pass a quarry on your left—likely used for materials to construct Lake Sherwood Recreation Area—before intersecting the Lake Sherwood Trail at 9.8 miles. Continue straight, again on the Lake Sherwood Trail. Retrace your steps over the spillway bridge, crossing the dam and returning to the trailhead, completing your loop at 10.6 miles.

Nearby Attractions

Lake Sherwood Recreation Area not only has trails aplenty but also a large lake with fishing and electric motorboating and paddling. Furthermore, it features a relaxing campground with a picnic area, fishing pier, swim beach, and hot showers.

Directions

From Exit 181 on I-64 at White Sulphur Springs, drive 15.0 miles north on WV 92 to Neola. From Neola, travel east on Lake Sherwood Road 11 miles and come to the recreation area. Pass the entrance gatehouse, take the first right, then make an immediate second right and head toward the picnic area. Follow this paved road to a circular turnaround with parking. The Lake Sherwood Trail and Upper Meadow Trail start here.

Blue Bend Loop

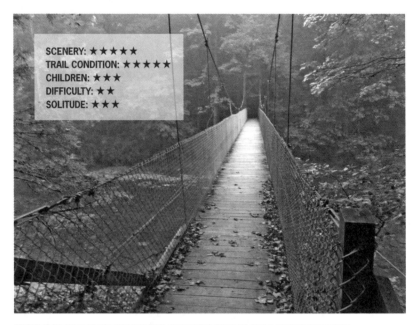

SCENERY: ★★★★★
TRAIL CONDITION: ★★★★★
CHILDREN: ★★
DIFFICULTY: ★★
SOLITUDE: ★★★

BEGIN THIS HIKE BY CROSSING THE SWINGING BRIDGE OVER ANTHONY CREEK.

GPS TRAILHEAD COORDINATES: N37° 55.275' W80° 16.029'

DISTANCE & CONFIGURATION: 5.3-mile loop

HIKING TIME: 3 hours

HIGHLIGHTS: Anthony Creek, Big Draft Wilderness, multiple views

ELEVATION: 1,900' at trailhead, 2,910' at high point

ACCESS: No fees or permits required

MAPS: *Big Draft Wilderness, Monongahela National Forest;* USGS *Anthony*

FACILITIES: Campground at trailhead, picnic area, restrooms, swim area, water spigot

WHEELCHAIR ACCESS: In immediate picnic area

CONTACT: Marlinton–White Sulphur Springs District, 304-536-2144

Overview

This loop takes place in the Monongahela's southeastern corner, at Blue Bend Recreation Area. Named for a nearby alluring swimming hole along Anthony Creek, Blue Bend also features a fine campground and picnic area in addition to the wonderful loop hike described here. The Blue Bend Loop Trail enters Big

Draft Wilderness, cruises along clear-and-pretty Anthony Creek, then climbs Round Mountain, where a trio of vistas awaits.

Route Details

This hike explores a lower, drier habitat than much of the Monongahela National Forest and is almost entirely within the Big Draft Wilderness, coming in at 5,144 acres. Established in 2009, it is the smallest federally designated wilderness in West Virginia, yet contains this fine loop, allowing you to explore the heart of it. If you can, plan to camp and swim at this special parcel of the Monongahela National Forest, in addition to making this excellent trail circuit.

Join the Blue Bend Loop Trail, leaving the corner of the recreation area parking lot. Pass through the picnic area shaded by preserved hemlocks to reach a huge swinging bridge over Anthony Creek. Climb it. Blue Bend, with its swim beach, is within sight upstream. You are about to follow crystalline Anthony Creek downstream. Reach the loop portion of the hike. Follow the Blue Bend Loop Trail right, heading downstream along Anthony Creek, a translucent mountain brook carving through a cliff-lined gorge. Sycamores border the watercourse, while rhododendron and other moisture-loving species flank the trail. Gunpowder Ridge rises tall across the creek, while Round Mountain reaches for the sky to your left. The trail runs along the creek, allowing you to glimpse into the stream, sporadically splitting around islands. Leave Blue Bend Campground behind and squeeze past a rock outcrop rising to your left at 0.4 mile. Look for trout and bass in the water. Find a deep swimming hole at 0.8 mile as stands of rhododendron find their place. Bisect a second flat before joining a woods track at 1.3 miles.

Meet the Anthony Creek Trail and Big Draft at 1.7 miles. The thus far–level Blue Bend Loop Trail turns left here and begins climbing the side of Round Mountain. The path switchbacks a steep slope, reaching a drier exposure where black gum, mountain laurel, pine, and oak rise amid scattered rock outcrops. Rock-strewn Big Draft flows well below, and will be nearly dry during summer and fall months. At 2.5 miles, the trail cuts through an evergreen-rich hollow before making the crest of Round Mountain. Keep working on your 1,000-foot ascent from Anthony Creek, reaching a trail shelter at 2.9 miles. This three-sided Adirondack-style shelter makes for a good break spot. The refuge's long-term fate is under question since the area is now a federally designated wilderness, making the shelter a candidate for removal. Water can be had from a spring below the shelter, though the spring may run dry in late summer and fall.

Blue Bend Loop

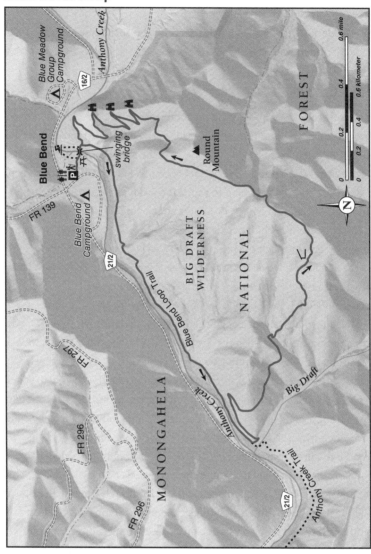

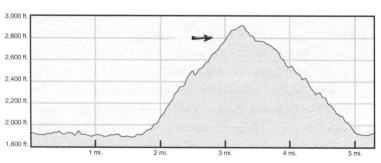

Leave the shelter, rising on a former roadbed. The trail widens as you shortly top out on Round Mountain at 3.2 miles. The walking is easy under open forest with sizable oaks. Watch for a hard left at 3.3 miles while descending, leaving the wide woods track for a narrow foot trail. Cut through a gap at 3.5 miles, then swing to the west side of Round Mountain, now on a prolonged descent. Anthony Creek flows far below. Cut through rhododendron thickets on the north side of Round Mountain. Come to a piney ridgeline and your first vista at 4.2 miles. This is a great place to linger and a well-deserved reward. Here, beyond the wooden fence, pastoral land and Christmas tree farms of the Anthony Creek valley open below. Coles Mountain stands to your right and Hopkins Mountain to your left.

The Blue Bend Loop Trail leaves the ridgecrest, switchbacking downward toward Anthony Creek. However, more rewards lie ahead, as the path returns to the ridgecrest a second time for another view in the same direction, but at a lower elevation, at 4.4 miles. The overlook here, 150 feet lower than the previous one, is bordered by a wooden fence. The switchbacks resume and lead to a third overlook at 4.7 miles, 140 feet lower than the last vista point. Leave the uplands for good via a final switchback, reaching the banks of Anthony Creek in gorgeous bottomland full of white pine at 5.0 miles. The trail meanders through the bottom, passing a large wooden and attractive waterside picnic shelter on your right. You may want to head over there and check out the Blue Bend swimming hole. In summer, it makes an idyllic posthike dipping spot. The path reaches the swinging bridge over Anthony Creek. Cross the span a second time, gaining a last view of the creek before completing the loop at 5.3 miles.

Nearby Attractions

Blue Bend Recreation Area features a campground, a swim beach, a picnic area, and a shelter. In addition, a restored fire tower keeper's cabin is a short distance up Forest Road 139, across from the recreation area entrance.

Directions

From White Sulphur Springs, travel north on WV 92 for 9.0 miles to Little Creek Road/County Road (CR) 16. Turn left on CR 16 and follow it 2.0 miles to CR 16/2 (Blue Bend Road). Continue forward on CR 16/2 and come to Blue Bend Recreation Area on your left in 2.0 more miles. Turn left here, then take your next left into a gravel parking area, with restrooms, before entering the campground. The hike starts in the right-hand corner of the parking area as you face the restrooms.

Appendix: Monongahela National Forest Contact Information

fs.usda.gov/mnf

SUPERVISOR'S OFFICE/FOREST HEADQUARTERS
200 Sycamore St.
Elkins, WV 26241
304-636-1800
One block east of US 219 at the Iron Horse statue in downtown Elkins

CHEAT-POTOMAC RANGER DISTRICT
Cheat Ranger Station
304-478-3251
On US 219 just east of Parsons

Potomac Ranger Station
2499 North Fork Highway
Petersburg, WV 26847
304-257-4488
1.5 miles south of Petersburg off WV 28/55

GAULEY RANGER DISTRICT
932 North Fork Cherry Road
Richwood, WV 26261
304-846-2695
1 mile east of Richwood on WV 39/55

GREENBRIER RANGER DISTRICT
304-456-3335
On WV 92/US 250 just east of Bartow

MARLINTON–WHITE SULPHUR RANGER DISTRICT
Marlinton Ranger Station
304-799-4334
On Cemetery Road off WV 39 at the eastern edge of Marlinton

WHITE SULPHUR RANGER STATION
1079 Main St. East
White Sulphur Springs, WV 24986
304-536-2144
On US 60 in White Sulphur Springs

CRANBERRY MOUNTAIN NATURE CENTER
304-653-4826
At the intersection of WV 39/55 and WV 150

SENECA ROCKS DISCOVERY CENTER
304-567-2827
At the intersection of WV 28 and US 33 at Seneca Rocks

Index

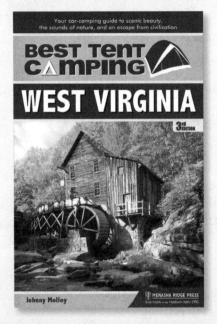
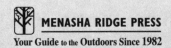

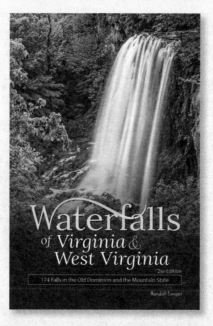

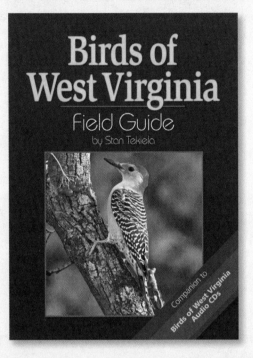
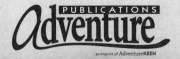

DEAR CUSTOMERS AND FRIENDS,

SUPPORTING YOUR INTEREST IN OUTDOOR ADVENTURE, travel, and an active lifestyle is central to our operations, from the authors we choose to the locations we detail to the way we design our books. Menasha Ridge Press was incorporated in 1982 by a group of veteran outdoorsmen and professional outfitters. For many years now, we've specialized in creating books that benefit the outdoors enthusiast.

Almost immediately, Menasha Ridge Press earned a reputation for revolutionizing outdoors- and travel-guidebook publishing. For such activities as canoeing, kayaking, hiking, backpacking, and mountain biking, we established new standards of quality that transformed the whole genre, resulting in outdoor-recreation guides of great sophistication and solid content. Menasha Ridge Press continues to be outdoor publishing's greatest innovator.

The folks at Menasha Ridge Press are as at home on a whitewater river or mountain trail as they are editing a manuscript. The books we build for you are the best they can be, because we're responding to your needs. Plus, we use and depend on them ourselves.

We look forward to seeing you on the river or the trail. If you'd like to contact us directly, visit us at menasharidge.com. We thank you for your interest in our books and the natural world around us all.

SAFE TRAVELS,

Bob Sehlinger

BOB SEHLINGER
PUBLISHER

About the Author

Johnny Molloy is a writer and adventurer based in Johnson City, Tennessee, who has been exploring the Monongahela National Forest for three-plus decades. His outdoor passion ignited on a backpacking trip in Great Smoky Mountains National Park while attending the University of Tennessee. That first foray unleashed a love of the outdoors that led the native Tennessean to spend over 4,000 nights backpacking, canoe camping, and tent camping since that time.

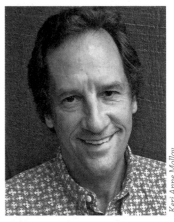

Keri Anne Molloy

Friends enjoyed his outdoor adventure stories; one even suggested he write a book. He pursued his friend's idea and soon parlayed his love of the outdoors into an occupation. The results of his efforts are over 80 books and guides. His writings include hiking, camping, paddling, and comprehensive guidebooks about specific areas, and books about true outdoor adventure throughout the Eastern United States, including several guides about Virginia's outdoors.

Though primarily involved with book publications, Molloy writes for various magazines and websites as well. He continues to write and travel extensively throughout the United States, endeavoring in a variety of outdoor pursuits.

A Christian, Johnny is a Gideon and active member of Christ Community Church in Johnson City, Tennessee. His wife, Keri Anne, accompanies him on the trail. Johnny's nonoutdoor interests include reading, American history, and University of Tennessee sports. For the latest on Johnny, please visit johnny molloy.com.